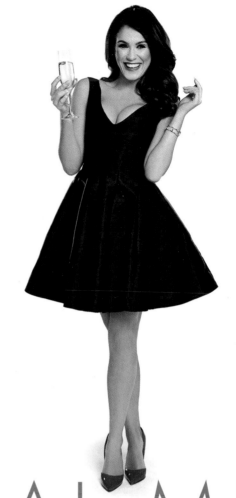

THE REAL ME

FASHION, FITNESS AND FOOD TIPS FOR REAL WOMEN – FROM ME TO YOU

Vicky Pattison

sphere

Contents

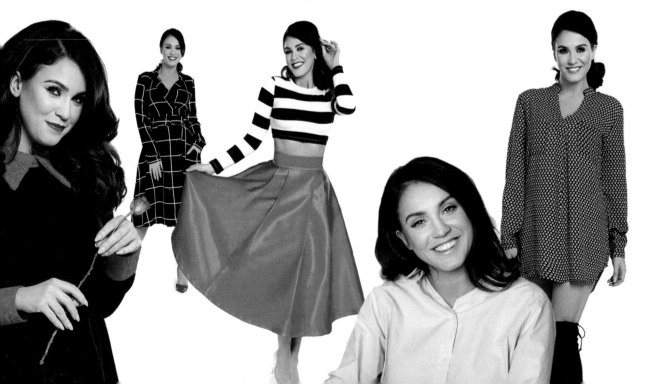

THE

FASHION, FITNESS AND FOOD

REAL

TIPS FOR REAL WOMEN

ME

FROM ME TO YOU

SPHERE

First published in Great Britain in 2016 by Sphere

Edited by Jordan Paramor
Principal photography: James Augustus
Additional photography: Brian Aris
For all other picture credits please see page 222
Designed and illustrated by D.R. ink

1 3 5 7 9 10 8 6 4 2

Important: Before starting any new exercise activity, discuss your plans with your doctor
to ensure any conditions specific to you are accommodated.

A CIP catalogue record for this book is available from the British Library.

ISBN 978-0-7515-6549-2

Printed in Italy

Papers used by Sphere are from well-managed forests
and other responsible sources.

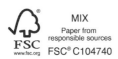

MIX
Paper from
responsible sources
FSC® C104740

Sphere
An imprint of
Little, Brown Book Group
Carmelite House
50 Victoria Embankment
London EC4Y 0DZ

An Hachette UK Company
www.hachette.co.uk

www.littlebrown.co.uk

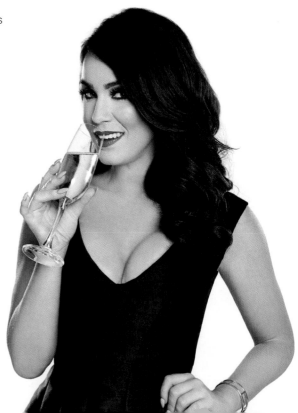

Highlights!

✳ If it's **embarrassing baby pictures** you're after, can I suggest you turn to page 13?

✳ Start on page 26 to find out about my **first-date fashion and beauty tips**, from the perfect outfit to **glamorous curls** (page 32).

✳ You know you want to read about my **worst fashion mistakes!** They start on page 55. You're welcome.

✳ If you think you you're too busy to work out, there are some **quick HIIT exercises** that you can fit into your packed schedule on page 78.

✳ All my tips for an amazing night out with the lasses start on page 82, including my **getting-ready playlist** (page 83) and **contouring tips** (page 89).

✳ Look at me pretending to be the sort of person who isn't always hungover on a Sunday on page 98, and learn how to make an **incredible detox smoothie** on page 101.

✳ Did you know I wrote a novel called ***All That Glitters?*** There's a sneaky free sample of the first chapter on page 125.

✳ If you want to get **bikini-ready for your hols**, you need my amazing **6-week gym programme** on page 137 – it'll get you into the best shape of your life.

✳ Break-ups are the worst, but one thing that will make you feel better is my incredible **brownie recipe** on page 168.

✳ I decided to let you **rummage in my handbag** on page 177. Yes, really.

✳ Did I mention I won ***I'm a Celebrity***? Check out page 196 for some of my favourite memories from the jungle.

✳ Nail your **winged eyeliner** with my step-by-step guide on page 208, and then turn to page 213 to **celebrate with 'The Vicky' cocktail**. (The next morning, you may want to refer back to page 108 for my **ultimate bacon sarnie**.)

About the *The Real Me* recipes . . .

I believe in eating healthily most of the time – I know I genuinely feel better about myself when my diet is on point. But I don't deprive myself; there are times in life when everyone deserves a naughty treat. So, 70 per cent of the recipes in this book are super healthy and you'll recognise them with this little angelic icon on the right. Each healthy recipe includes information about its nutritional benefits and is the type of meal or snack I *try* to eat as part of my daily diet. They're all delicious – that's a **Vicky Pattison guarantee** – and I hope they inspire you to try something new.

The rest of the recipes are for those moments when only sweet treat or a cheeky cocktail will do. Of course, they come complete with their own devilish symbol! No nutritional benefits – let's just enjoy them and not feel guilty about it!

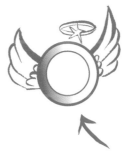

Super healthy!

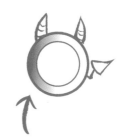

No guilt please – just enjoy!

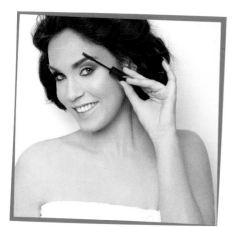

And a little note on make-up!

I am very lucky to work with lots of lovely make-up artists who use all sort of amazing products on my face. All the make-up tips and tutorials in this book include the high-end products that they use to make me look half-decent in front of the camera, and which over time I've added to my own make-up bag. But we've also included incredible alternatives that do the same job brilliantly, but won't break the bank. The high-end products are always **highlighted in a colour** and the high-street alternatives are **highlighted with this elegant grey**, so you can find them easily!

This book is dedicated to everyone who has ever had a dating disaster, a fashion fail, a make-up mishap or a cooking catastrophe . . . join the club!

This is my chance to say that I'm not perfect by any stretch of the imagination, and that like every other human being I make mistakes.

I make fashion mistakes, I make make-up mistakes, sometimes I don't get my hair right, and I've been known to have very embarrassing fake-tan fails. And let's not get started on my love life! (We will, don't worry.) But over the years I've picked up loads of different tricks that help me to look better, feel better and – most importantly of all – strive to *be* a better person.

Looking back, there've been times when I wish there had been someone there to give me a bit of a helping hand and pass on advice when I was confused about life, love and hangovers.

Some of the stuff in this book may seem obvious and some of it may not seem that logical, but trust me, it will make sense at some point. I've done an awful lot in a very short space of time and I've been lucky enough to learn a lot of lessons from both my slip-ups and my successes. I'm also very fortunate to have loads of amazing and very talented people around me, teaching me new things every day. All of the beauty tips, recipes and exercises in this book have been passed on to me by the people I work with every day: the make-up artists who I have heart-to-hearts with at 8 a.m., as they try to make me look human before I go on TV; the personal trainer I've been working with for years, and who knows just how hard I've worked to take control of my health and fitness. I learn so much from them, and they've all become my friends. I couldn't do what I do without them, and now I want to pass on some of that wisdom to you.

Ultimately the mistakes I've made have helped me to become the person I am today. I'm finally proud of myself and I'm happy with who I am inside and out.

I want every woman in the world to feel like that, so here's a really simple piece of advice to kick the book off.

If you ever have down days or you're feeling insecure or unsure, please just remember this:

YOU'RE AMAZING!

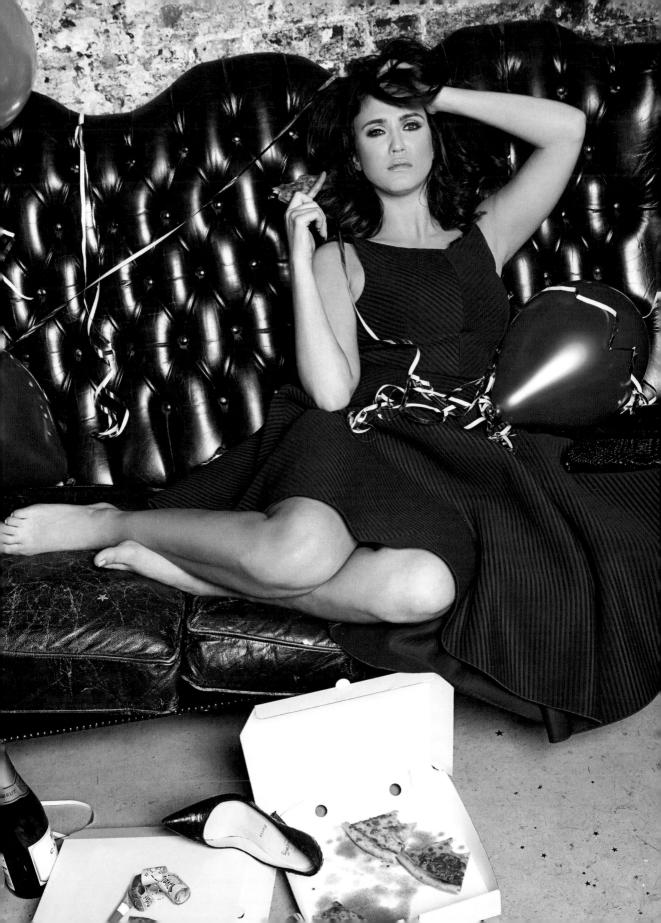

HOME IS WHERE THE HEART IS

Why I'll never forget where I came from.

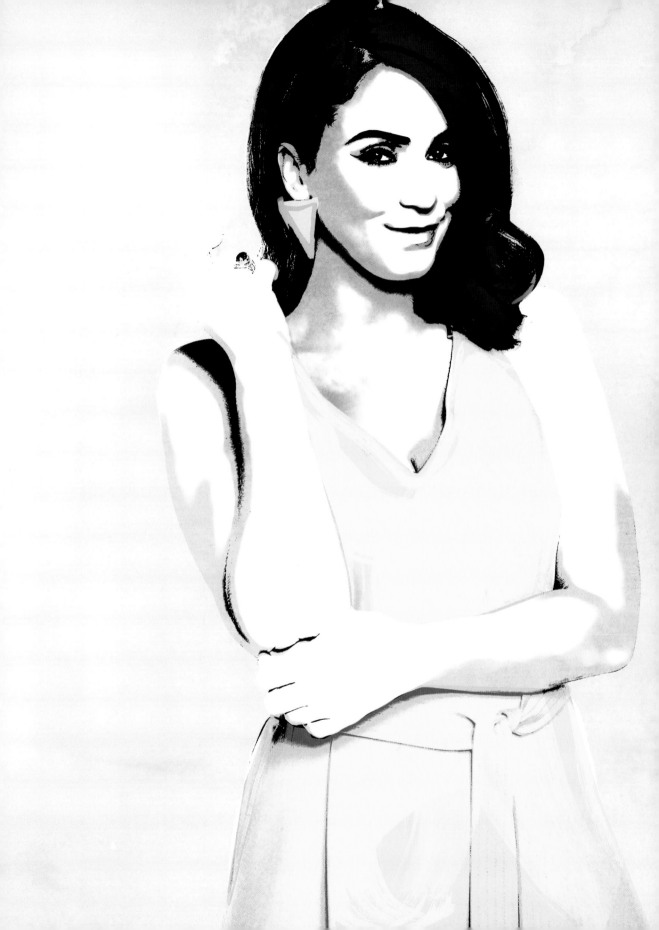

Where it all began (and some really embarrassing photos)

If you've read my autobiography, Nothing But the Truth, *you'll already know a bit about my younger years. But I could talk about my friends and family all day, and I want you to get a feel of what it was like for me when I was growing up in Newcastle.*

It's my favourite place in the world, and I will never forget my roots. My home, my friends and – most of all – my family have made me who I am. They know the real me.

Meet the Pattisons

I had a very normal, humble start in life and I can't fault the way my mam, Caroll, and dad, John, brought me up. They did everything at the right time, and because they were so settled I always felt content. I think these days so many people rush into relationships because their friends are doing it or because they want a kid before a certain age, but my parents weren't like that at all.

My mam and dad went to the same middle school, The Buddle in Wallsend, which still stands today. My mam fancied my dad but he was really shy so *she* pursued *him*. I think that's where I get my feisty, go-getting attitude to blokes from. My dad thought my mam was out of his league and would never have dared to try and chat her up. Mam knew that, so she kissed him. That was when she was fourteen, and they started properly going out when they were fifteen. They were engaged at nineteen, married at twenty-four, had me at twenty-nine and my sister Laura at thirty-three. They did everything in their own time, in their own way. They weren't pressured into anything and their hand was never forced.

They wanted to live together before they got married, so they did, even though it was kind of frowned upon back then. My mam has always impressed on me how important it is to really get to know someone before you settle down, so there are no surprises. She always says you never really know someone until you live with them, and she's dead right. That goes for friends and boyfriends too.

Mam and Dad even had their wedding their way. Back then it was traditional for people to get married in the morning, but my mam didn't want to feel rushed so they did it at 3 o'clock. My dad had been out for his stag do the night before and he'd fallen over drunk and hit his head on a mantelpiece! He was so worried about looking bad in their photos . . . I'm sure Mam was *thrilled* with that!

Even after they were married, they still had their own lives and they would go out with their own mates separately, which was quite unusual for couples back then. They were definitely ahead of their time! They marched to the beat of their own drum; they were together for ten years before they even thought about having kids because they had things they wanted to do.

They were always off on holiday with their mates and they've told me hilarious stories about their adventures. One time they were driving home from a night out with my auntie Ann and uncle Ross, and my auntie Denise and uncle Peter, when the bottom completely fell off their car. Five of them were hammered and the one sober designated driver had to deal with it. It sounds like something out of a *Carry On* film!

When I came along, Mam and Dad were properly settled and ready for family life. They were living in their third house, which was the one I grew up in until I was fifteen. Dad was working in the civil service, which he did right up until he retired, and Mam was looking after me. She said that if she turned her back for a minute I'd be up to all kinds of mischief. She's got the brilliant photo of me where I had covered myself head to toe in Sudocrem while she was busy making my lunch.

Mam couldn't have loads of time off after having me so she went back to work and often did several jobs at once. She worked in the office at a big industrial company called Ingersoll Rand, then she joined the civil service with my dad, and after that she had all sorts of jobs. She did book fairs and she was also a telephone canvasser – I've always said I get my work ethic from her! But even though she and Dad were very busy, they always made sure they had loads of time for us kids.

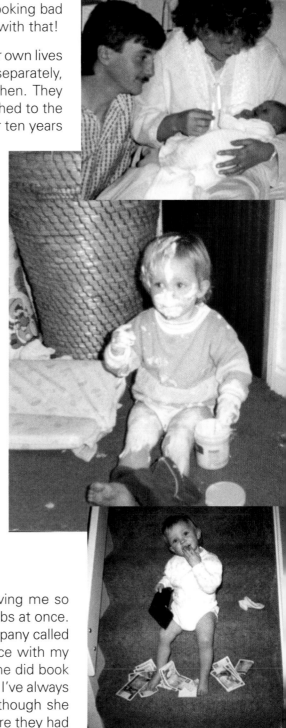

Girls just wanna have funds!

Before I was born, my dad had really wanted a boy, and even after I came along he used treat me like a little lad, dressing me in shiny shell suits so I looked like a small parachute. One day when I was about five, my mam had to go to work and I was in desperate need of a haircut so she asked my dad to take me. She was driving home later when she saw his car parked outside our local barbers. She pulled in and spotted me sitting in the chair about to be given the Kevin Keegan mullet my dad had requested. Needless to say, Dad never got asked to take me for another haircut!

Sometimes when he was looking after me, Dad would tell Mam he'd taken me to feed the ducks. Only he hadn't taken me to the park; he'd taken me to the pub with him and his mate who was *called* Ducky. He'd buy me a packet of Hula Hoops and I'd throw them at Ducky to see if he could catch them in his mouth!

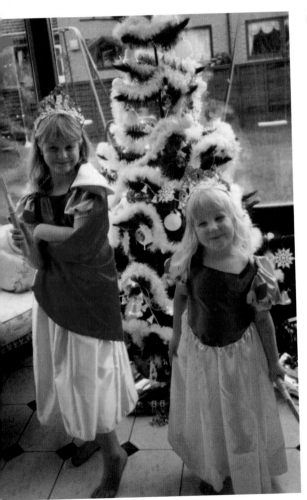

Queen Victoria and Princess Laura. I was regal from a very young age.

Sister act

I have a really clear memory of finding out I had a sister. I was only three, so I didn't truly understand what was going on and what a monumental impact this little baby was about to have on my life. Laura was born in the middle of the night and my dad phoned to tell us straight away. I remember my gran waking me up and saying: 'You've got a little sister!' I don't think I truly understood the implications of it, but I was excited because they were and my gran, granddad and I held hands and danced around to celebrate.

Once I met Laura, I was so in love with her. I used to hold her and squeeze her all the time; I thought she was perfect. But of course things changed when we got older. By the time she was about three we started to fight like cat and dog and she once bit the inside of my thigh so hard it bled because I wouldn't let her play with one of my dolls. To be fair, we had a perfectly normal sibling relationship!

But while we could fight and call each other anything we wanted to, no one else could. I was fiercely protective of her. I remember the first Christmas after Laura joined my primary school. We were doing a big nativity show where I was playing the innkeeper, which made me furious because I only had one line. (I've always been an attention seeker!) Because she was one of the tiny ones, Laura was an angel. One day in rehearsals, our teacher asked for the 'group one' angels to go up on stage. All the kids apart from Laura ran up on stage – she knew she was group *two*, but she had been left behind on her own. She was only four and she got really upset and started to cry.

I saw one of the other staff walk up to our teacher and tell her there was a little girl crying. She replied: 'I know. I'm trying to ignore her. That sound she's making is distracting everyone.' I was absolutely *fuming*, because I knew Laura had done the right thing – and even if she hadn't, she was only a baby. I stood up, threw my innkeeper staff to the side and ran off the stage and over to hug Laura. I told my mam when I got home and she went up to the school and gave the teacher hell. That teacher will always rue the day she ever messed with one of the Pattison sisters.

I always looked after Laura at school, but as soon as we were back home we'd be at each other's throats again. She always wanted to play with my friends, but I hated her hanging out with us. I wanted to be a grown-up with my older mates and instead I had this little 'mini me' following me around.

Me, Laura and Mam.

Our relationship changed a lot when I went to uni. Laura was getting more grown-up and when I left home we started to properly miss each other. We'd always been under each other's feet and we didn't realise how amazing it was having each other until we were apart.

I can't get enough time with Laura now. She's just the best thing and we're so close.

Going to uni was a massive turning point for me generally when it came to my family. I don't think I'd appreciated them enough and once I was away I realised how much they did for me and how lucky I was. They had put up with a lot from me for the past eighteen years and I missed them terribly.

Squad goals

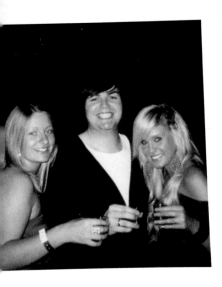

Me and Burnsey with our friend Alex, back in the day.

I've had a lot of the same friends for years and years now, and I think the world of them all. I've hung out with the same group of fifteen girls (and one guy called Burnsey!) from back home since we were in our teens and while we've changed over time, our friendship hasn't.

As time's gone on and my life's taken me down south more permanently, I see my old gang less than I used to. But it's a true testament to our friendship that we're still as close as we ever were. I always think that with a true friend you don't have to see them every day, but when you drop back into each other's lives it's like you've never been apart.

I met most of those friends when I was about fifteen or sixteen and I started going out in town and getting Saturday jobs. I met my friend Kailee when I worked in the shop G-Star in Newcastle; I met Steph because she worked in my favourite nightclub, Blue Bamboo, and Paul – aka Burnsey – used to be the host in TGI Fridays. I thought he was super cool because he got to welcome all the guests and be the 'face' of the restaurant.

I've had some of the best times of my life with that group. We used to go out on a Friday and not get home until Monday and we'd have such a laugh. Obviously we can't do that any more because people have got grown-up responsibilities. We're all in different places in our lives: Kailee is about to have her second kid, my friend Zoe from uni is getting married and Lindsay's buying a house with her boyfriend in Leeds. We're quite spread

> **I always think that with a true friend you don't have to see them every day, but when you drop back into each other's lives it's like you've never been apart.**

out, but we still make sure we get together for birthdays or other special occasions. No matter how busy I am or where I am in the country, I will always make time for them. When there's an event coming up I'm the first one to say: 'What are we booking?' and I'll get it sorted. We may not be able to party all weekend like we used to, but we still find loads of ways to have fun together. We'll go bowling, or we'll go to someone's house for pizza and gossip. The activities we do have changed, but the way we feel about each other hasn't. And actually when we're together, we want to be able to catch up on each other's lives and that's hard to do if you're mortal in a loud club. But having said that, we still have some bloody great nights out on the lash together.

I'm sure some of them probably don't understand my life choices – and vice versa! I can't ever imagine settling down with a couple of kids, but equally they probably wouldn't enjoy what I do. I think our ambitions and the difference between what we want out of life has never been more obvious, but still we totally support each other and always will.

Another reason they're my best mates is because they still treat me just the same as they ever did. I've been out for dinner with 'new' friends I've met

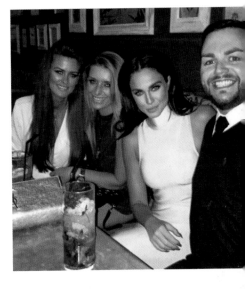

over the past few years and when I've offered to pay the bill, they've let me. I'm happy to treat my friends, *of course*, but if I offer to pay when I go out with my lot from back home they're like: 'No way. Put your money away.' That's how I know they love me for *me* and they don't expect me to put my hand in my pocket all the time just because I'm earning more money than I used to. To them I'm still the same girl who had to live on Pot Noodles because I'd spent all my wages going out with them at the weekend.

Some of my best friends ever (Gemma, Sarah and Burnsey) on a random weekend back home.

We're all very like-minded and they would never let me change. They will always be such a special group to me. We get each other and we love each other. We've been through so much, from working abroad together to going through break-ups and marriages. We've seen things go wrong and things go right, and no matter what happens I'll still be the same Vicky to them, and I wouldn't change them for the world. I couldn't be prouder of any of them.

That's what friends are for

What matters to me when it comes to friends is that people have my back and they care about me. To me, good friends are people who don't take themselves too seriously and who you can totally be yourself around.

A good test is to gauge how you feel when someone rings you. Do you look at their name on the phone and think 'I can't answer that', or do you look and think 'I don't care if I'm really busy, I've got to take this'? You can always make time for the people you truly want to make time for.

You have to surround yourself with people who make you feel good, because they're the ones who will bring out the best in you. Friends should make you the best possible version of yourself. If they don't, something's not right. Life is way too short to spend hanging around with people who don't make you a better person in some way.

Every time I see my lasses I know there will be gossip and drama, and maybe some tears – but I love all of that. I like girls' girls who like spending time with other women. I can't stand it when someone is hanging out with you but looking over your shoulder to see if a nice lad is coming in the door. No way. If you're on a girls' night out, lads take second place.

If I meet a girl my age who doesn't have a serious group of girl friends, it's a massive red flag to me. If you're a woman who can't get on with other women, it makes me wonder what you've done. I like women who support each other. When I saw my friends after I won *I'm a Celeb*, they all told me they voted loads and they cried when I won. They were so happy for me. Not one of them showed even a hint of jealousy. That's what being mates is all about. You build each other up and you take pride in your friends' achievements.

I get so much pleasure from my friends doing well, I almost feel like it's me achieving what they have. Too many people are out for themselves, so they're bitter and jealous when people do well and I don't want any of that in my life. Those people only hurt themselves.

I love funny, loyal, strong women who aren't afraid to say what they think.

I also love girls who love a good night out and love to party. When my mates and I would go out for nights out when we were younger, we were like a pack of wild hyenas and we stuck up for each other and put on a united front if anyone said anything nasty about one of our group. Obviously we've grown up a bit now and we're calmer in the way we defend each other, but that fire is still there and I think you have to have that. Disloyalty is a guaranteed way for me to lose interest in someone. It doesn't take me long to detach if I don't think someone is loyal. I also can't stand by someone who isn't showing me respect. There is no friendship without respect.

When you're younger you can overcomplicate friendships and your life revolves around who does and doesn't like you and which of your friends are and aren't getting on. But friendships shouldn't be complicated, and as you get older there are bigger things to worry about. If someone makes you feel good, makes you laugh and you walk away feeling amazing and knowing you've had a great time with that person, that's a true friend.

I'm still at the stage of my life where I enjoy going out partying and I've made new friends along the way who are at similar stages to me. People like my friends Gavin Foord, Alex Cannon from *Judge Geordie* and lovely Casey

Batchelor and Cami-Li. Like me, they're living their lives without strings and it's nice to be able to have the best of both worlds.

I know it's a bit of an obvious thing to say, but I do have to be more careful with my friendships now. I know I can trust all my old friends one hundred per cent, but I have to tread carefully when it comes to letting new people in. It's hard because you come across people who want to use you in all walks of life and more than ever in the entertainment business, and that concept is so alien to me. It's astounding to me that anyone would actively seek a person out because of what they can do for them. It's not because of their personality or because they're interesting to be around or they're fun; it's because they think they can get them somewhere. I cannot for the life of me work that out.

If someone comes up to me being nice, I take them at face value and think they want to get to know me because I'm funny or I've got something to say for myself. But it's taken me an awfully long time to get my head around the fact that some people have an agenda. Whoever it is, whether it's a boyfriend, a friend or even somebody you don't know that well, it will never stop being hurtful. Someone is effectively saying that who and what you are is not enough and they want more from you. I've been burnt a few times over the years. Finding out people have sold stories on me is the worst thing. Especially because instead of getting annoyed with them I get frustrated with myself – because I don't learn.

But having said that, do I really want to learn? Do I want to be so hardened and bitter I see every person as a threat? No, I don't. Instead I've decided to keep my naive, wet-behind-the-ears approach to everything and take everyone at face value. If they're not genuine they'll be found out at some point anyway, and I don't want to end up going on a one-woman crusade to weed out the bad people in the world because I have better things to do with my time. I want to spend my life focusing on nice people and try to see the good in everyone. If that means I still get burnt every now and again, then so be it.

I can't let the people who have hurt or disappointed me in the past affect the way I look at new people, because then they've won. The entire human race isn't bad and I don't want my experiences to make me sceptical about life. We're all just human beings and sometimes we make mistakes, and I can't make a handful of idiots accountable for everyone I'll meet in the future because I'd be doing myself – and them – an injustice.

I think what makes me a good friend is the fact that I'm loyal, protective, fun, generous, compassionate and not quick to judge. Friends often come to me with their problems because they know I've probably done worse!

My friends always say they like the fact that I'm always up for a party and a laugh and I try not to take things too seriously. And there's nothing I wouldn't do for someone I consider to be a friend. *Nothing.* I would go to the ends of the earth for them. If I'm your friend, I'm your friend for life.

I'm not one of those people who will talk behind other people's back either, and I never give the impression that it's okay for someone else to do it to me. People know they can't be two-faced around me. It you don't like someone, that's fine, but if they're my mate don't be slagging them off to me, thank you very much.

Not everyone's cup of tea

I think as you get older you become more comfortable with the fact that you won't like everyone, and not everyone will like you. When you're younger, you see it as a bit of a failure if you're not best mates with everyone in the world, but the simple fact is we're all different and sometimes people clash. It doesn't mean you have to have a big row with anyone you don't like either; just let it be.

I certainly went through a stage where I used to argue with people I didn't get on with, but part of being a grown-up is learning to live and let live. If you walk into a clothes shop you're not going to like everything in there, but that doesn't mean you have to be mortally offended by a dress you dislike and start having a row with it. You just move on and find one you do like.

There's actually a massive sense of relief once you realise it's okay not to be universally loved. I don't know what the turning point was for me but I know that for a while I was really angry and defensive and I almost didn't *want* people to like me. Or I didn't really give them a chance to, especially during the *Geordie Shore* years when I felt like everyone was judging me anyway.

I stopped caring how I presented myself to people because I felt like they'd already made up their minds about who I was. Then I had a word with myself and realised that I was just cementing my bad image by being really angry about it.

I've actually got a lot fewer friends than I had a couple of years ago, which I think will surprise people. Actually no, that's not true; I've got fewer *acquaintances* than I had a couple of years ago, but I've got a hell of a lot more friends. My circle has got smaller but I've still got the same amount of solid mates.

Leaving *Geordie Shore* and meeting some great new people made me feel more positive and happy, and that had a knock-on effect on everything. I decided that if I was nice to everyone, and I smiled, they couldn't help but be nice back, and ninety-nine per cent of the time that's true. And if someone does snub you, it says a hell of a lot more about them than it does about you.

I realised that if I was good to other people, it would come back on me tenfold and that totally changed my outlook on things. The people around me changed because *I* did. I stopped being scared of not being liked and learnt to be liked for who I am. I'm just myself now and if someone thinks I'm okay that's great, but if you don't, nay bother pet.

I would rather be a few people's shot of tequila than everybody's cup of tea.

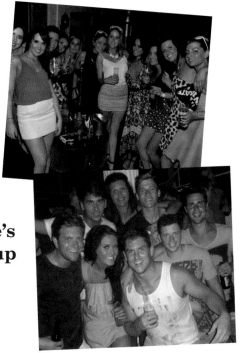

Top: *Me and the girls in Marbella for Kailee's sister's hen do.*
Bottom: *Ibiza with the lads!*

THE DATING GAME

Learn from my mistakes, ladies!

2

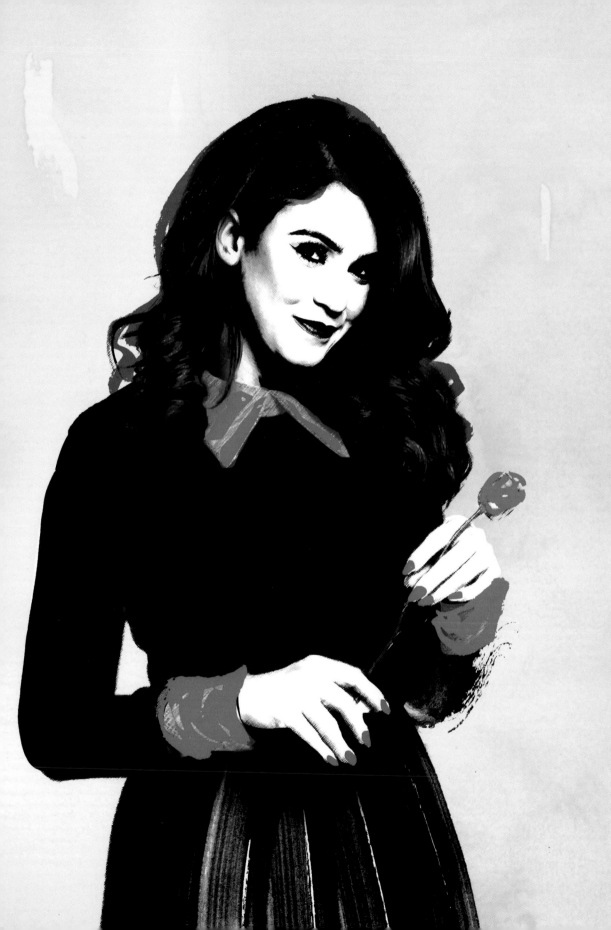

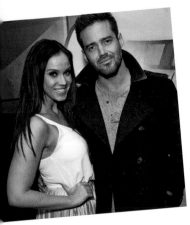

Hot date

Dating is one of my absolute favourite things, and when you're young and single I think it's important to go on plenty of dates to meet lots of different people and have a few adventures. A friend of mine once said that dating is a little bit like going into a sweet shop. You might know that your favourite sweets are strawberry laces, but that's not to say that you don't also like flying saucers. And sometimes it's nice to have a cheeky bar of Galaxy or some Tangfastics.

In short, variety is the spice of life and just because you like one thing that doesn't mean you might not enjoy another. Don't create a fantasy man in your head, who is so 'perfect' that you never give anyone else a chance.

Having said that, I do believe in 'the one' and I hope that when I meet him the whole room is going to stop. I want everything to descend into a blur and all I'll see is him. But in the meantime I don't think there's anything wrong with dating Mr Right Now.

My dos and don'ts of dating

Do

✓ Spread your wings. Don't be afraid to date outside of your comfort zone or social group, because you never know who could be right for you.

✓ Be confident and always **be yourself** on dates.

✓ What you want! Don't feel as if you have to see lads other people expect you to. I hate it when people judge people for having 'lots of boyfriends' or going on lots of different dates and trying to work out what's right for them.

✓ Be honest.

✓ Treat people how you want to be treated.

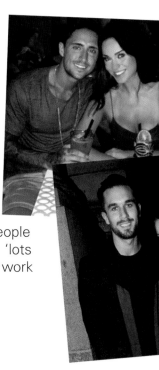

Don't

✗ Play games with people or be cruel, because it will come back on you.

✗ Two-time people. I won't pretend I haven't done silly things in the past, but it's never been intentional.

✗ Be the other woman. Remember, if they do it for you, they'll do it to you as well.

✗ Try and change someone. You *can't.*

✗ Try to be someone's saviour. A person has to want to save themselves. It's not your job to fix anyone's life and you have to embrace other people's faults.

✗ **Settle**. Never be with someone for the sake of being with someone.

How to look incredible on a first (and hopefully second . . .) date

First dates are an exciting and nerve-wracking time – and, let's be honest, they're also the time when you're going to put the most thought into what you're wearing! You can say what you like about only being interested in someone's personality, but the truth is that first impressions count and the confidence boost you'll get from looking good will go a long way to help you get over those first-date nerves.

I read that someone will form an opinion about you within three seconds of meeting you, so as shallow as that sounds, the truth is your date's going to be looking at how you present yourself. You'll get a second date based on what you say, but you'll impress at the beginning of a first date because of how you look.

You want to look amazing, of course, but you also want to feel comfortable. There's nothing worse than constantly feeling like you have to pull your top up so your boobs aren't hanging out, or yanking up a pair of ill-fitting jeans. If you feel confident and you feel sexy, you're going to put your best foot forward and that will shine through.

If there's a certain body part you're proud of, that's the bit to show off. If you've got good arms, go sleeveless. Your boobs and legs don't need to be out in order for you to look sexy – why not flash a little bit of collarbone in a strapless dress? I'm not one of those people who thinks, 'No one's going to buy the cow if you give them the milk for free'. If you want to show skin, show skin! You're only young once. I'll flash my back or a little bit of cleavage or my abs, but I'm very careful not to do it all at once. There's no need. You don't want everything to be out there. You have to leave something to the imagination!

The key is to make the most of what you love. Because I like my waist, my go-to outfit at the moment is a cropped jumper or a little top with a prom-style midi skirt because it's cute and it's sexy, which for me is the perfect look for a first date.

There's no point in wearing something you've seen on the front page of *Vogue* if the only person it suits is Cara Delevingne. If you don't feel relaxed it will be written all over your face. It will seep from your pores, and there are already enough things to make you feel nervous on a first date. Your outfit shouldn't be one of them. Embrace who you are. Embrace your body shape and *own it*. You got that first date for a reason so be nothing other than yourself. If you want to wear jeans, wear jeans. It doesn't matter as long as you're happy.

Date outfit triumph

I recently had a date with a guy I'd been out with before, but hadn't seen for a really long time. When we were together the first time around, I was so into him that I was constantly nervous and trying to be sexy and funny so he'd like me too. That resulted in me not being myself and not really enjoying

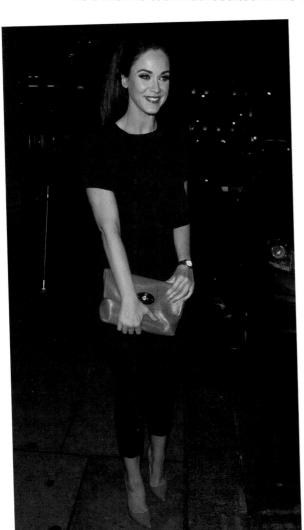

dating him as much as I should have. When we revisited the relationship, it was essentially like going on a first date again. But this time I *knew* he liked me because he'd come back a second time. So when the time came to go on the date, I was feeling really confident.

I mulled it over and in the end I just wore a very plain black jumpsuit, a red bag and shoes and red lipstick. I put my hair up very simply and I felt great. My entire outfit was high street apart from my Mulberry bag, and I felt really happy and that made a brilliant night even better.

A black jumpsuit is one of my favourite looks because it's quite figure-hugging but it's not in your face. I think classic colours are good for a date too.

I love a bit of monochrome with a red lip. I don't think you can go wrong with it.

Date outfit tragedy

My worst date outfit has to be when I went on my first *ever* date with my first *ever* boyfriend, Dean. I thought I looked super cool in my orange cargo pants, Caterpillar boots, a little belly top and an oversized parka. I looked like I was in All Saints and Blazin' Squad at the same time. I haven't got a photo of the outfit sadly, but if you look up pictures of Kenzie you'll get an idea.

How to create the perfect make-up base

A first date is like foundation . . . it's the base you build everything else on. (Do you see what I did there?) Lame jokes aside, there's no point going all out on

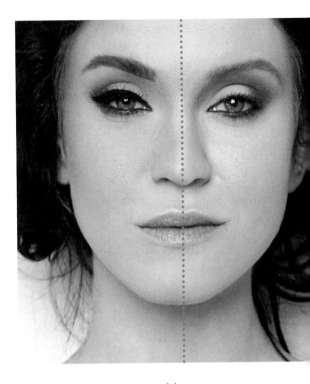

your outfit if your make-up doesn't cut it. This picture shows me with one half of my face completely made-up (except for lippie!) and the other with only the base and eyeshadow – you can see what a difference a bit of slap makes! Over the course of this book, you'll see how to add in all of the different elements to make up the whole face: the contouring (page 89), a red lip (page 91), the brows (page 106), and flicked eyeliner (page 208). And to see me with no make-up on at all, turn to page 195! Let's start at the beginning here with the building blocks of the whole thing: the base.

(**Top tip**: if you know you're a bit messy when it comes to doing eye make-up, you can easily switch around the order and do eyes first. That way you're less likely to mess up your base!)

✳ One life-changing tip I've picked up from make-up artists is to ensure that my skin is properly exfoliated before I apply a base – this helps achieve a perfect, smooth finish. The Clarisonic handheld cleansing brush is incredible – it's an investment as you buy the device and just recharge and change brush heads. It magically buffs all the dead skin cells off when used just twice a week. It beats any exfoliating cleanser creams, but if you don't have time then a great quick alternative is a simple exfoliating wipe!

✳ The perfect base provides the canvas for all your other make-up, so it's worth taking time on.

✳ I always use a moisturiser to start with, and I make sure I leave plenty of time for it to sink in before putting anything on top.

✳ I'll then pop on **Smashbox Photo Finish Foundation Primer Pore Minimizer**. It's oil-free and gives my skin a matte look. **Maybelline Baby Skin Instant Fatigue Blur** does a similar job. You don't want to be putting foundation on if your face feels even slightly greasy. (If you have dry skin, you probably don't need a primer and your moisturiser will do the job on its own.)

✳ Next I'll add concealer under my eyes. If I've had a late night, I'll neutralise the dark shadows with a peach shade either from **Bobbi Brown's range of correctors** or **NYX Dark Circle Concealer**. I then layer **NARS Radiant Creamy Concealer in Custard** lightly over the top. (**Collection's Lasting Perfection Concealer** is an amazing alternative for this.) On a good day, the NARS on its own will be enough, but if I still need a bit of help then **MAC Prep + Prime Highlighter Light Boost** is the last element, to further brighten if needed. Try **L'Oréal's True Match Touche Magique** for a similar effect.

✳ I'll then apply **Too Faced Born This Way** or **Revlon's ColorStay** foundation all over the face with a **Real Techniques Setting Brush**, avoiding the eye area. You'll ruin the effect of your concealer by layering foundation over the top. You want to blend the foundation into the under-eye concealer, but try to avoid overlapping.

✳ I'll set my foundation and concealer with translucent powder before I go on to contouring. I usually switch between **NARS** and **MAC powders**, but **GOSH's Velvet Touch Primer & Setting Powder in translucent** is also amazing. **MAC Studio Fix** used with a powder brush (not the sponge it comes with) is great for a little bit of extra coverage and keeping things in place for a long time. **Kiko's Weightless Perfection Wet and Dry Powder Foundation** will do the same job brilliantly.

✳ Once that's all done, I might give myself a spritz with **Urban Decay All Nighter Long-Lasting Setting Spray**. I hear that lots of girls use hairspray to set their makeup . . . Stop and use this instead!

✳ Now I'm all good to move on to the rest of my face . . .

Date outfit inspiration!

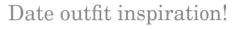

I really like denim in
general because it can
be sexy and casual at
the same time.

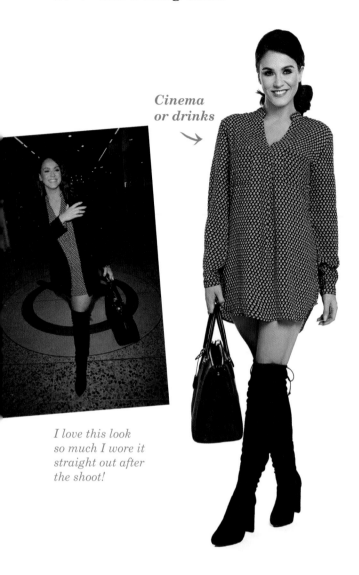

*Cinema
or drinks* →

*I love this look
so much I wore it
straight out after
the shoot!*

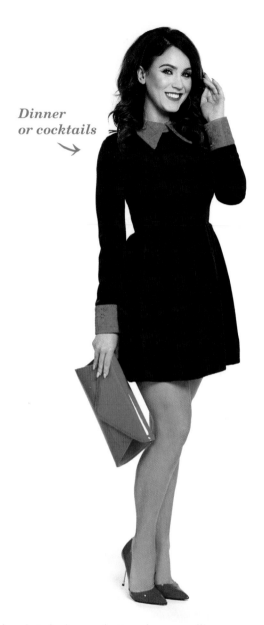

*Dinner
or cocktails* →

If you have one of those days when you're not feeling your best and you want to be comfortable, a shirt dress is perfect. You can still have your legs out and be flirty and feminine, but you're not feeling restricted in a tight pencil dress. You can also whack on a pair skinny jeans or leather trousers with it and change the look completely. This would be great for midweek drinks after work – effortlessly sexy.

I absolutely love skater dresses like this one – they're really sweet and sophisticated. Because this has got a high neck and long sleeves, you can get away with a slightly shorter hemline. The little flashes of red mean you can have red lips and red shoes too – my favourite combination!

A perfect date outfit for dinner in a nice restaurant.

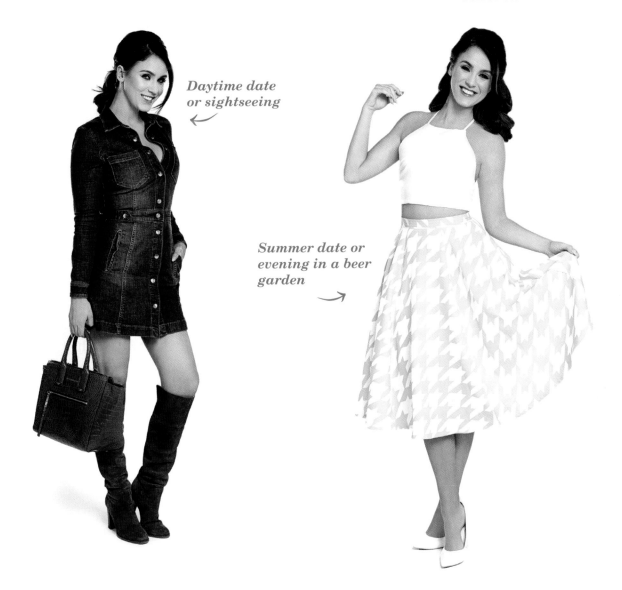

Daytime date or sightseeing

Summer date or evening in a beer garden

I really like denim in general because it can be sexy and casual at the same time – however you dress it up, you're never going to look like you're trying too hard. And the knee-length boots and bag pull the look together. I'd wear something like this for a daytime date – in fact, I wore something very similar on a trip to Harry Potter World recently! It's also perfect for a boozy weekend lunch with the girls.

This look is very summery and perfect for sitting by the river or having a few drinks in a beer garden. I don't wear an awful lot of pink and this is probably the 'girliest' thing I'd go for, but I think the houndstooth print makes it slightly edgier. The strappy top is great too – you're not showing too much flesh, but you're flashing a cheeky bit of midriff.

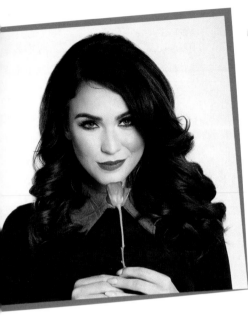

The fuss-free way to get long, loose curls

✳ I love curls because they're completely timeless and they can make even the simplest outfit more glamorous and show you've made an effort.

✳ I start off by applying L'Oréal Elnett Heat Protect Styling Spray. It's really lightweight but it smooths the hair out so you can get loads of volume. I'll use that to pre-prep my hair and then blow-dry it.

✳ The biggest mistake girls make when they're doing their hair is overdoing it with heat appliances. Prepping the hair is the most important thing. If you don't blow-dry your hair properly before you set a style, it will just fall out.

✳ Do your blow-dry with a big round brush so you're already manipulating the hair into a natural curl. If you dry it straight, you won't have much bounce or lift. Get as much body and bend in the hair as you can.

✳ I'd recommend doing a set of pinned up curls while you're blow-drying. Take sections of hair that are roughly as big as you want the curl to be – the bigger the roll, the bigger the curl – and create loops. Start from the top and roll downwards so you elevate the hair as you do it. That way you'll get a natural root lift. If you do it from the bottom you'll end up with flat roots, which equals flat hair.

✳ You could also use a set of tongs to create individual curls and secure them in the same way. So you tong, pin, tong, pin – but make sure your hair is completely dry before you do this.

✳ Secure each curl to your head with a grip and repeat until all of your hair is curled in the same way.

✳ Leave the curls in for as long as you can (if you've used the tongs, wait until the curls feel cool to the touch) and then take them out and use your hands to loosen the curls out from the roots.

✳ You've now got a good platform to work from and you can either leave the curls quite tight, soften with a wide-toothed comb to create waves, or even brush the curls out so your hair has just got a delicate, soft movement in it. All of these things will make sure you don't end up with an overly 'set' finish.

✳ Long, loose curls work well with both extensions and natural hair, but you need to keep your extensions in good condition. They don't get the natural oils from your head so the best way to keep your extensions in good shape is to use a leave-in conditioner on them. Something lightweight works well. If you use anything too heavy it will drag it down. You can also apply a bit of oil on the ends if they're feeling dry. But only use a tiny bit because you don't want it looking greasy.

What the dates I've been on have taught me (and I've been on quite a few)

I think it's good to feel nervous before a date because it shows you're excited. But it's also important to remember that whoever you're meeting is just another person, and if it doesn't go well it's not a reflection on you. If he's not right, you can dust yourself off, get a Domino's with the girls and slag off his shoes.

I like going for drinks on a first date because I think it's the best way to have a relaxed conversation. Avoid the cinema, because you don't get a chance to talk, which may seem like a good way to side-step awkward chat, but it won't help you in the long run. Save the cinema for five or six dates in, when you want to do the whole 'snuggling up' thing. Drinks can make you feel more relaxed, and a bit of social lubrication never hurt anyone. Just don't get smashed. (Rich coming from me, I know!) I would recommend you stop at three drinks. Four at the very most. Don't get hammered and make a helmet of yourself, tell him you love him, spill a drink on him or start crying over your ex, all because you had a few too many gins!

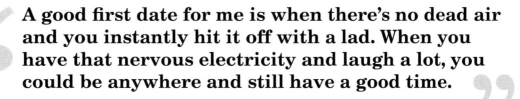

A good first date for me is when there's no dead air and you instantly hit it off with a lad. When you have that nervous electricity and laugh a lot, you could be anywhere and still have a good time.

If you're quite a confident person you can always go for food, but I think a meal can be really daunting on a first date. I've been for dinners where I was really self-conscious about eating in front a guy and even chewing made me nervous. I think that's a perfectly understandable fear. Dinner might be a better choice about three dates in, when you're feeling more comfortable and it's not going to be a massive disaster if you dribble Bolognese down your top or get a herb stuck in your tooth.

Find the date style that's perfect for you. If you like to have a couple of drinks to feel comfortable, go to a bar. But if you want to have a laugh try go-karting

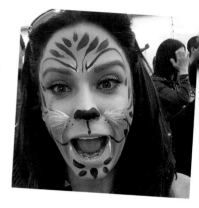

or even Spanish dancing. Being on *Ex on the Beach* taught me how brilliant unusual dates can be. It may be a bit embarrassing at first but nothing breaks the ice as quickly as you both having to get to grips with some sort of crazy activity – it takes the focus off your nerves so you can relax and have fun.

I love dates that are different. I like trying unusual stuff and I love it when a lad shows initiative. Similarly, I think most lads love it when girls take the lead. Dates where people think outside the box are so much fun and it will make you remember them. One of my best dates ever was when I got taken to London Zoo, and the lad I was with suggested we got our faces painted. I was a tiger and he was a lion and we walked around like that all day. We laughed, we ate ice-creams and we had a brilliant day. Don't be afraid to embrace your inner child and have fun.

Get yourself on Groupon or Wowcher and see what they've got to offer because you can get some brilliant deals for things you'd never normally think of doing. You could do a river cruise or horse riding on the beach and end up having one of the best days of your life. Even if you never see the guy again, you'll have had a laugh and tried something new. I once bought a sausage-making course on one of those sites. (It's a long story. I'd had a few wines . . . oh, actually it's not that long – I was drunk!) Imagine if you took a geezer sausage making! Whatever happens, it's a good conversation starter and if they don't 'get' it they're not the one for you. I'm not saying sausage making is for everyone, but something like that can really separate the men from the boys, or the cocktail sausages from the Frankfurters!

I'm not going to lie; I love being wined and dined and I'm quite traditional in that sense. There's nothing nicer than a man putting on a lovely suit and taking you out to a nice restaurant. Someone took me to The Oxo Tower once and I felt like a princess. Those kinds of dates are so lovely. Having said that, I also think that in this day and age if we're demanding equal everything we have to open our eyes to the fact that a man might want to be treated like a prince occasionally, and there's nothing wrong with that. I have no problem with organising where we're going and picking up the bill.

Relationships are built on equality, respect and trust, and you only get out of them what you put in. It's amazing when you're made to feel special, but remember that your lad might like a bit of that back too. Please don't be that girl that never offers to buy a drink, that girl is a knob.

I will offer to pay on a first date, but I do think maybe that's when a lad is trying to impress you so nine times out of ten he'll probably say no. A first date is a special time and it sort of sets a precedent. So if he's strong and he respects you, that's when he's going to show it. And if you do the same and you show you're bringing something to the table – even if it's just getting a round in – that says a lot too.

Swipe right?

I've never tried internet dating but I'm certainly not saying I wouldn't ever do it. A business partner of mine is moving in with a girl he met on match.com soon and they're so adorable and well-suited, and I've heard a lot of other similar success stories. Another friend met her lad on Tinder when he came to her town on a stag do and they're really happy too. I think love and compatibility can be found anywhere. You don't have to meet someone through the traditional routes of being introduced through friends. Technology is better than ever so we may as well take advantage of it. The science behind how some sites match people is incredible, and a world away from spotting someone across a bar and thinking they're a decent bit of kit.

If you're on a website or an app you can find out the things it's too awkward to ask in real life. Like, does he want kids? You could get six dates in with someone before you realise that they're ten years younger than you or they've already been married three times or they want eighteen kids. Online dating may not feel like the most romantic or natural way to meet someone, but you have all the information you need in front of you and I don't think that's such a bad thing.

Subjects to avoid on a first date if you want a second one

You want the conversation to flow on a first date, so don't make it awkward by opening up about anything and everything to the point where it makes things uncomfortable.

Never talk about exes on a first date. *Ever.* It's tempting to try to make yourself sound really desirable by saying that your ex is obsessed with you or something, but it just makes you sound like a bit of a twat. Equally, if you and your ex parted on bad terms, your potential new lad does not need to know about it.

Don't ask questions you don't feel ready to know the answer to. There is stuff you should get to know organically about a person, like their dating history. Imagine how intimidated you'll feel if they blurt out they used to date a Victoria's Secret model.

Don't ask anything too intimate, or reveal your deepest, darkest secrets to him after a few drinks. You might end up never seeing this lad again, so do you really want him walking around with all this knowledge about you?

First date chat should be light and fun. I always try to talk about holidays or music or nights out and if the date is right that could kick off a really good conversation.

If the banter doesn't flow, be realistic about the fact that it's probably not going to work.

If you don't want to see the guy again at the end of the date, chances are they're probably going to be feeling the same. If they don't it could be a bit awkward, but honesty is always the best policy.

If they text you afterwards and ask to see you again, be as polite and considerate as possible and say something along the lines of, 'I had a good time and you're a great guy but I don't see it going anywhere. Sorry, but I'd rather be honest.' Telling little white lies to protect someone's feelings doesn't make you a liar or a bad person. If anything it makes you quite sweet.

Learning the hard way

The truth is, you have to learn the dos and don'ts of dating the hard way. And I certainly did that on one of my first ever dates. I went on a night out with my mates, got really drunk and met this guy I thought looked like David Beckham. I

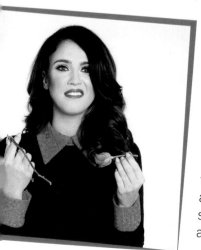

gave him my number and he texted me the following day. I'd already disco-tashed him in the club and my mates assured me he was a total rocket, so I decided I must have liked him and figured I had nothing to lose.

We arranged to go out for drinks and to the cinema the next night at The Gate in Newcastle, which is the height of sophistication when you're 17. This gorgeous dark-haired guy walked through the door and I thought, *Bloody hell, Vicky! You've smashed it here. He's some sort!* But he walked straight past me and into a bar. Gutted. Then I turned around and there was this gangly, unfortunate-looking geezer standing in front of me. He smiled and said: 'All right, Vicky?' . . . and I just thought, *Nah.*

I felt too bad to leave so I followed him upstairs to the cinema and he went to get the tickets. When he came back he had one cinema ticket in his hand and he said: 'I've got my ticket and I'm in seat J23 so you should get seat J24.' Seriously. We went to get a drink before the film started, and when he went up to the bar I took my opportunity to leave. I got into a black cab outside and went home without looking back. I still feel a bit bad about it and I would never do something like that now!

The 'L' word . . . and all the rest

You should never compromise on a relationship and you should never accept anything other than the real thing. I have no notion of loving someone by halves and I don't want to have.

I don't understand these people who get into a relationship and can't be bothered to see the person they're with. One of my friends moans about arguing with her boyfriend every time I see her and I don't understand why they're still together. They don't have any ties to each other so I really want her to find someone who makes her happy.

Love should be mad and passionate and boot the face off you, not half-hearted. I don't mean having rose petals sprinkled on your bed every day, I'm talking about getting butterflies when he sends you a text and holding hands and kissing when you're walking along the street. You should care about that person more than anyone else. There is nothing better than when you have that crazy mutual respect for each other and not only fancy each other, but also find each other really funny. There's nothing better than that feeling of not wanting to go to sleep because sleeping feels like you're leaving someone.

The worst relationships I've had are when people try to change me. What you see is what you get with me. I'm fun, I'm feisty, I'm opinionated, I'm driven and I won't let you get away with any BS. I work hard, and I value my friends and family above everything else. If you want to be in my life you have to accept that.

I will be madly, passionately in love with someone, but I'll also be busy getting on with my own stuff; I'm not the sort to sit around waiting for someone to finish work and have their dinner on the table. I won't be waiting up for them when they've been on a night out because the chances are I'll be out later. A lad has to be all right with the fact that sometimes they won't be able to see me when they want to, or that sometimes I'll want to pay for dinner.

I'm upfront with guys about this. I don't steamroller them with a ton of information all at once but I do let them know what they're letting themselves in for. I don't pretend to be this ditzy idiot who is going to laugh at their stupid jokes and make them feel like the big tough guy.

A lot of guys will claim they're looking for a strong, independent woman because the idea of it is sexy, but the reality is that not many men can deal with it and they quickly become childish and stroppy – or worse, angry. The hardest thing for me is when guys like the idea of me, but they don't like the reality of having a girlfriend who doesn't take any crap. I don't think you should ever try to change someone in a relationship. If you don't like who they are, don't be with them.

Remember who you are

You should never let someone tell you what to do in a relationship, and you have to have trust. It's lovely when you want to be around someone, but you shouldn't be in each other's pockets constantly. You still have to have your own life.

Never allow yourself to be defined by a relationship. My biggest fear in life is that I'll just become known as someone's girlfriend, as if I'm a plus one. Never be someone's 'and'. Being in a relationship can be so lovely but don't ever lose your identity.

At the moment a lot of girls I know around my age are settling for the wrong people because they have some kind of desperate need to settle down. I don't know if they feel pressure from society or if they feel like their biological clock is ticking. Or maybe it's because their mates are doing it? Never rush into something with the wrong person because you want the situation. I know people who have had kids with the wrong geezers just because they want kids. Or they're buying houses with blokes because they want to live with someone. Or they're getting engaged to a twat because they want to be married before they're thirty. Why the rush? It's a million times better to take your time and be with the right person rather than just any person.

No one is putting these ridiculous restrictions on you apart from yourself. Relax, take the pressure off and don't be with someone because you don't want to be alone. Ultimately, you'll end up feeling lonelier and unhappier.

Don't treat a relationship like it's the 2 a.m.–3 a.m. power hour in a club, where you have to find someone to neck on with before the night finishes or you'll have to try to pull someone in a kebab shop. Don't scramble for a five out of ten just so you don't have to be on your own. (Although sometimes I have the best part of my night in a kebab shop, if you catch my drift.)

You have to have faith. There are so many things you can be enjoying in your life. You can be going out on dates or hanging out with the girls and having a laugh, or forging forward with your career. A serious relationship and a man is not the be all and end all. Have a bit of chill and don't allow pressure to influence what you think you want.

I will hold my hands up and admit that some of the blokes I've been out with were total tossers. But I've never been out with someone just so I have someone to cuddle up to on a Sunday. I would much rather be on my own and happy than coasting with the wrong person.

Relationships can be tough sometimes. In the beginning it's fresh and new, but then the reality of everyday life kicks in and things stop being as special or exciting as they were, and you just have to roll with it. You have to accept that you're not going to be on cloud nine every single day, and you need to focus on all the good things. And remember that no matter how happy and loved up couples look on Facebook, no relationship is perfect and everyone has their problems to overcome.

I think the best thing to do if you're single is to not actively look for love, but be open to the prospect. And in the meantime, have a different kind of fun because there is so much freedom in being single.

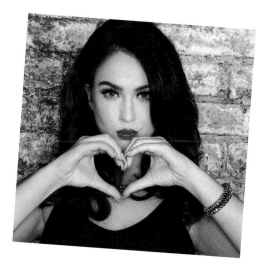

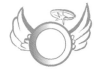

The way to a man's heart . . .

Once you're into the swing of things (and you've got over the eating-in-front-of-him anxiety), a surefire recipe for dating success is inviting your new bloke round for a romantic dinner. I'm no expert in the kitchen, but even I can manage this one!

Middle Eastern lamb with hummus courgettes (*serves 2*)

Ingredients

For the hummus courgettes

3 courgettes

½ tub (100g) hummus

⅛ cup plain, live yoghurt

½ tablespoon lemon juice

Olive oil

For the lamb mix

½ tablespoon olive oil

½ medium onion (diced)

250g lamb mince

1 teaspoon cumin

25g pine nuts

½ tablespoon thyme leaves

On the side

250g broccoli florets

Method

1. Preheat the oven to 200° C.

2. Prepare the courgettes by slicing them in half lengthways and scooping out hollows from the flesh, using a small spoon or melon baller.

3. Mix together the hummus, yoghurt and lemon juice in a bowl and set aside.

4. Meanwhile, heat ½ tablespoon olive oil in a large frying pan over a medium heat and add the onion. Fry for 5–10 minutes or until the onion is soft.

5. Add the lamb mince to the pan, breaking up the chunks, and brown for approximately 8–10 minutes. Add the cumin, pine nuts and thyme, and fry for a few more minutes.

6. Add 125ml water to the pan and bring to the boil. Reduce the heat, cover with a lid and cook for 15–20 minutes.

7. Meanwhile, rub the courgettes with a little oil and place on a baking tray (hollows facing upwards). Bake for 10 minutes.

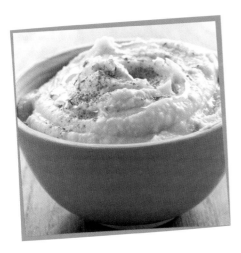

8. Remove the baking tray from the oven and fill each courgette half with the hummus mix. Return to the oven and bake for a further 10 minutes.

9. While the courgettes are baking and the lamb is cooking, steam the broccoli until tender. If the lamb has finished cooking, it can be kept warm with the lid on and the heat turned off.

10. Once everything is cooked, lay 3 courgette halves in a row on each plate. Divide the lamb mixture evenly over the courgettes on each plate.

Benefits: *Topping courgettes with the lamb and hummus mixture boosts your vegetable intake whilst keeping starchy carbohydrates low.*

Hummus is made from chickpeas, which are a great source of phytoestrogens for a healthy hormone balance, as well as a host of minerals such as zinc for immunity and manganese for metabolism and blood-sugar control.

This dish is ideal if you have guests with food intolerances as it is naturally gluten- and dairy-free.

MISS INDEPENDENT

How to survive in the big bad world,
all by yourself.

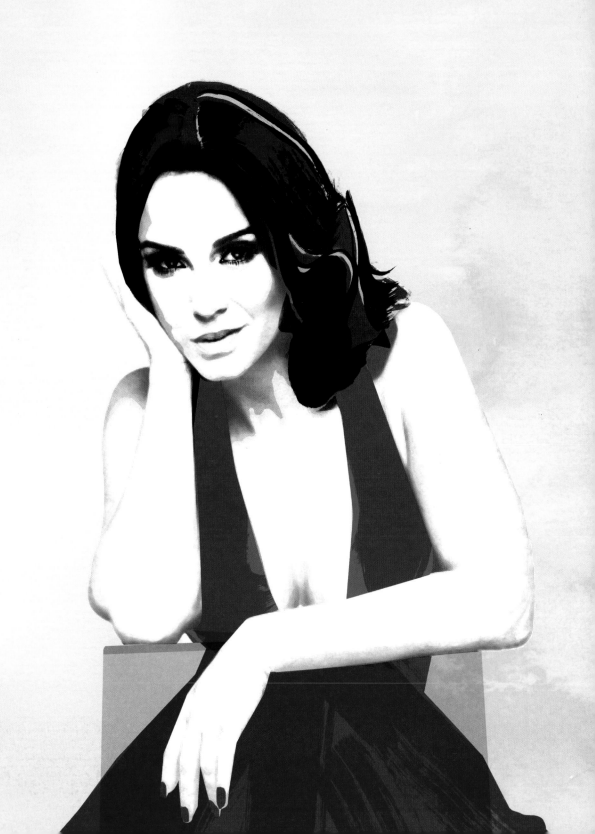

How I did (and didn't) handle leaving home

Moving out of home is a massive step for anyone. It's the first time you learn to stand on your own two feet, and whether you move out to live with the girls or a boyfriend, or you go to uni or do a season abroad, it's a huge, huge deal. I didn't realise just how much my mam and dad did for me until I actually left home. You suddenly have things to pay for that you've never even considered before – like gas and electricity, and even food – and that you've always taken for granted. You have to learn to budget pretty quickly and it's such a big responsibility.

Flying the nest

I was lucky in a way because I kind of dipped my toe into being away from home before I moved out properly. After I did my A-levels, I headed to Magaluf to do a season and I worked in a bar called Boomerangs on the strip for three months. It was so wicked. I moved into an apartment with five other people who were also working at the same place. It was a two-minute walk from the beach and work and everyone I lived with was really fun.

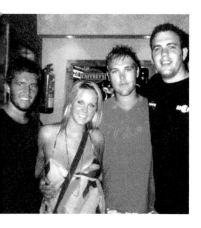

Me and my Magaluf lads.

Every Friday I gave 70 Euros to my friend Kim, who ran the apartment, and that covered my rent, our cleaner and bills, so I didn't even really have to take care of that side of things. All I had to do was feed myself. It was all really exciting to me. I felt like I was standing on my own two feet but I had a huge safety net below me if the ground gave way, and that was knowing I would be going back to the family home at the end of the summer.

After Magaluf I went to uni, which was a whole new level of independence. I was committing to living away for three years, which felt like a very long time. Also there was no holiday vibe like there had been in Magaluf! You weren't moving around and meeting loads of new tourists constantly. At uni you couldn't bail out and not pay your rent and hope your landlord didn't find you on the strip. You were committed to a course, and unless you dropped out completely, you had to commit fully.

I chose my uni courses on my mam's advice. She said to me: 'I know you don't know exactly what you want to do, but if you don't do something you like you won't go, so choose what you enjoy.' And it was as simple as that. I chose cities that I wanted to live in with bright lights and good nightlife, and I picked drama and media courses that sounded varied and exciting.

There's a saying that goes, 'If you do something you enjoy, you'll never work a day in your life'. It's the same with education. If you choose something you like, when it comes to busy times and dissertations you won't feel so much like you want to do a Usain Bolt-style runner.

Even at uni I wasn't completely self-sufficient. When I got my student loan it all went on fees and housing so my mam would put £65 into my account every Friday. She could have essentially given me a £3,500 loan each year, but she drip-fed it to me because otherwise it would have gone within the first month. I didn't have the common sense not to spend it on ridiculous things, and I don't think many 18-year-olds do.

To bulk up my income I worked in Kookai, and I also sold shots in bars because I wanted to keep living the lifestyle I'd become accustomed to in Newcastle. I wasn't your average student wearing the same pair of jeans for weeks and no make-up. I went to uni in Liverpool for God's sake. I used to get a blow-dry, fake tan and my nails done every Saturday!

That £65 from my mam was a godsend. Kookai paid monthly and I earned around £300 a month there, so by the time that came in I'd end up spending it on something I really wanted, like a nice new going-out outfit or a big night with my mates.

I had a desire to work hard and look after myself instilled in me from a young age, and being at uni taught me how to work even harder and budget for food and travel. There was no one to get me out of bed in the morning and make me go to lectures, so that was all down to me too. I had proper responsibilities. Having said that, I think I only ever went to about three Thursday morning lectures because there was a night know as Medication at a club called Nation on a Wednesday night and it was my favourite place to party. Medication is the reason I know so little about the history of theatre!

But for the most part, I had to properly manage myself, and that meant my lectures, my homework, Kookai and doing the shots on a Friday. Most of the friends I knocked about with worked at the Student Union or promoting club nights, but they were more like bit jobs to get in a few quid, because a lot of them had extra loans from their parents. That's why my mam gave me my extra money; she was very mindful about other people having more than me, and she didn't want the fact I had to earn money to affect my uni experience.

The problem with me is that, unlike a lot of the other students, I didn't want to dress in cheap clothes. I still wanted to have a nice pair of shoes from Faith, and me and my friends wanted to go out for nice meals. If it was one of our birthdays we'd do something like go and get tickets to see Girls Aloud at the MEN arena and get a table at Mansion in Manchester. We weren't your usual 'go down the pub in your trackies' students. We were glamorous Liverpool students. That was the life I wanted, so I was happy to work for it.

That whole period was a great life lesson for me. It taught me that if you want something or you want to live a certain way you have to be willing to get your head down and work for it, because nothing will be given to you. Uni also taught me how to manage my time, and I learnt to juggle a lot of different things.

I also learnt a lot about myself and about how to be respectful when you're living with people. My flatmates and I had so many arguments about those really clichéd things like who drank the last of the milk, and I never thought I'd be that person. To be fair, it was usually me who had done it, but over those three years I at least learnt to replace it if I did.

The best advice I've got for anyone who's thinking of moving out of home is to only do it when you're ready. Looking back I probably went a little bit too soon. I was, and still am, the most independent woman in the world, but I still struggled with my first year of uni. My mam says that's because I only had one night back home after Magaluf to prepare for Liverpool and mentally I wasn't ready.

I didn't land on my feet at all when I first arrived in halls. I think you're either really lucky with the people you live with or you get totally stitched up, and sadly it was the latter for me. I lived with one girl who was doing a PE degree

> **The best advice I've got for anyone who's thinking of moving out of home is to only do it when you're ready.**

and was very serious about it. Another girl was from Southport, which is only an hour away, so she went home all the time. I also lived with a girl who didn't drink, and another one who stayed in her room with her boyfriend all the time. All in all, it wasn't ideal.

I remember being so excited about going to Freshers' Week events, but not one of the girls I lived with was up for it and I really struggled with that. I was doing a joint honours as well, so that was another punch in the dick. I was trying to divide my time between two courses so it was hard to make friends there too.

Homesick blues

I was homesick from the moment I arrived and it took me months to settle in. Homesickness is very real, so if you're suffering talk to someone about

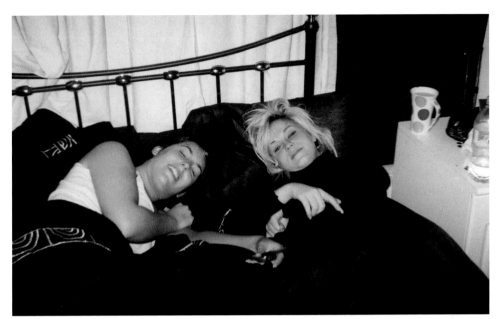

Recovering at uni after a night out at Medication.

it because a lot of other people are going to be in the same boat. We don't always have all the answers ourselves, and someone else might be able to help you. And don't feel ashamed because you don't instantly feel completely self-sufficient just because you've left home. At the end of the day you're only a few weeks or months older than you were when you lived at home and your mum still did your washing, so don't feel like you have to morph into a fully rounded adult overnight.

I nearly gave up and went back home a couple of times because of my homesickness. I'd gone from being this big fish in a small pond in Newcastle, where everyone knew me and I was never more than five minutes away from a friend, to a place where nobody knew me and I didn't know anyone. I had expected to have people high-fiving me the minute I walked into the Student Union. I thought it was going to be like *Hollyoaks* and everyone was going to be desperate to be my friend. But it's not. You have to essentially start all over again and it's scary and it's hard work. The thing you have to remember is that everyone is just as petrified as you are, they just might not be showing it.

My saving grace was a lad called Liam who I'd lived with in Magaluf. By complete coincidence he went to Liverpool too, so I started hanging out with him and his mates a lot. If it hadn't been for him I would have been sitting in on my own every night, as miserable as hell. One night Liam asked me to go along to a mixer in the Student Union. I was quite nervous but in the end I made loads of friend really quickly and things totally changed for me after that. If he hadn't given me that push it could have been a very different story.

I still maintain now that I should have done the season in Magaluf and then gone back home and got a job in Newcastle for a year before I went away again. Or maybe even done the summer season earlier, or the following year. Basically, I should have done it any other way than the way I did because the transition was too quick and I was left feeling so anxious and miserable I very nearly gave uni up.

Please don't feel obligated to go to uni just because you're 18 and you *can*. Just because your mates are all going it doesn't mean it's the right time for you. So many people get shepherded in and they get carried along with what everyone else is doing because society or other people say it's what they should do. I think people should think long and hard before taking that leap and you will *know* when it feels like the right time.

The same applies to leaving home for other reasons. A friend of mine once moved in with her boyfriend simply because she'd been with him for two years and he asked her. She felt like it *should* be the obvious next step, even though she was really happy living at home at that point. It ended in disaster because she was pissed off about having to deal with boring stuff like bills and making her boyfriend dinner. She was still really young and she wanted their relationship to be exciting, and the everyday things got in the way. In the end they split up and the next time she moved in with a boyfriend she made sure it was for the right reasons and not because of pressure.

When you feel like quitting, think about why you started

After a rocky start I ended up meeting some of my best friends at uni, so I would say always give things a proper go if you think there's a chance it could work out. If you hate it and it's making you really down, get the hell out of there. But if you think there's hope, give it a good shot. Quitting is not in my nature, and if I'd quit before I'd given it a proper chance I would never have forgiven myself.

I used to go home and see my family as much as possible, and that was actually quite detrimental to me in a way because all I was doing was running away from my problems. But I did get the advice and love I needed. I'd have a night out with my mates and tell them about what a crap time I was having at uni and they would say: 'You like it here because you're only back for the weekend, but you'd be bored to death if you were back here full-time with nothing to do and no direction.' And they were right. My only other option at that time was moving back home and getting a full-time job there, which would have driven me mad.

After a weekend back home I'd return to uni with this renewed sense of vigour and purpose, knowing it was what I wanted and also aware that I'd have to put in more effort if I wanted to make more friends. I knocked on doors and I chatted to whoever I could, and by the first Christmas I was friends with everyone who lived in the flat above me, as well as loads of other people.

By the end of my three years in Liverpool everyone knew my name and it became like a second home. It made me realise feeling uncomfortable is all about growth. If you stay in the same lane and go at the same speed all your life you won't learn and adapt and become a better person. I grew so much at uni and I'll always be so grateful for it. Especially the difficult parts because they propelled me forward.

Although I missed Liverpool a lot when I left, it felt good to be back home. I'd missed my family and it was nice to be looked after again. The only problem was I'd got so used to being able to do what I wanted, when I wanted to do it. At uni I could go and come as I pleased, play my music as loud as I wanted to, and leave things in a mess and no one cared. But my mam and dad weren't quite as laid back as my housemates had been and I had three years of them saying to me: 'You treat this house like a hotel.' And they were right.

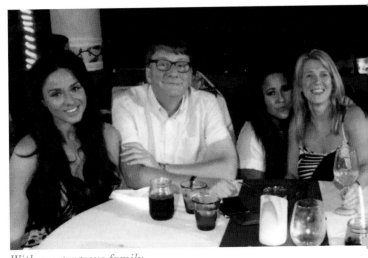

With my gorgeous family.

It was a very testing time for my relationship with my mam. I thought I was a lot more grown-up than I was. I was striving for adulthood but not quite getting there because I was still living under my mam's roof. I wanted to have control over my life, but of course my parents wanted me to be respectful because it was their house. It was difficult to take that step back and be told what to do again, but I wasn't in a financial position to live on my own at that time.

I get on brilliantly with my family now but that was a tricky time. I was very lucky they were so understanding but I could probably have made it a lot easier on myself by not acting like I was still a student!

My style evolution

My style has completely evolved from when I was younger. And to be honest, it needed to. Some of the things I used to wear are shocking.

When I was younger I could never have imagined myself wearing a dress with a high neck and collar, but as you get older you find out what works for you and now I love tea-dresses because they suit my shape.

One thing I will never wear again are hot pants. Literally *no way*. There was a time when they were super cool because Girls Aloud were wearing them all the time, and my mates who had long skinny legs looked great in them. But sadly I did not have the legs for them. Or the arse. They were a bad move for me and I'd like to leave that look firmly in the past. If I turned up on a date now wearing them, I would fully expect the lad to do a runner.

When it comes to fashion you have to be aware of your strong points and blindly following trends isn't going to get you anywhere. If something isn't right for your body shape and you're wearing it more for someone else's benefit than your own, you're not going to feel good.

Back in the day my friends and I thought that in order to get a bloke's attention we had to be wearing practically nothing, but now I cringe thinking about how I used to be constantly pulling down short skirts. I must have looked so fidgety and uncomfortable. I'm not about that any more. These days I go for a mixture of style and comfort.

My signature style now is quite classic. I love that whole glamorous, old Hollywood vibe. But at the same time I'm still in my twenties and I don't mind doing a bit of experimenting sometimes. I like to be feminine and I'm not one of these women who's into the androgynous look. Maybe that's because my dad made me dress like a boy until I was seven?

I like to follow trends to a certain extent, but I like to put my own take on them. Just because I've seen Kendall Jenner looking great in a mesh jumpsuit on a catwalk it doesn't mean I'm going to rush out and buy one, because the chances are it won't look the same on me. That's fine because I'm not a supermodel and what suits her won't suit me. But you can adapt things. I don't necessarily like myself in skinny jeans because my thighs are my least favourite bit of my body. That's why I think a denim dress or a longline denim shirt is a nice alternative for me. They're not emphasising a part of my body I've got a hang-up with. Always emphasise your best bits and play down any you don't like.

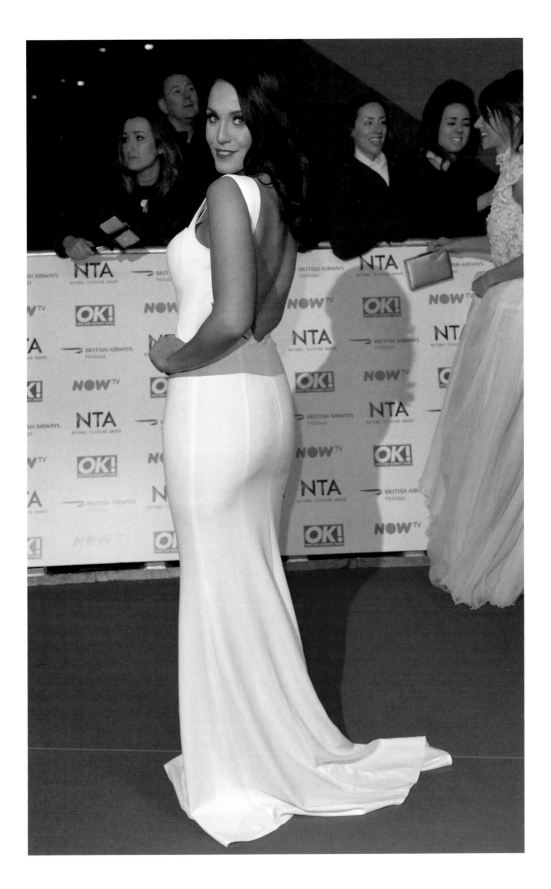

Making friends with the sale rail

Fashion-wise, things were hard for me when I went to uni because I didn't have an awful lot of money to spend on clothes. I'd gone from living at home and spending all of my spare money on new outfits, to having to buy bin liners (not to wear).

I hate sales but I had to find ways to make my money go further so I started shopping in them all the time. I remember buying this dress from Miss Selfridge that had gone down so many times in the sale I got it for £1. It was a blue backless jersey dress and I wore it until it fell apart.

Because I still wanted to buy nice things, sometimes I saved money in other ways. I was friends with people who worked in bars so I got free or cheap drinks, and I'd let them use my Kookai discount in return. I became very resourceful. I got a lot of student cards to save money on all sorts of things, and I got a Young Persons Railcard, which saved me a fortune on trips home.

I used to share wardrobes with my housemates too, and all of my clothes got a lot of repeat wear. I had some nice bits from when I lived at home, and some stuff my mam had bought me, but everything else I got cheap. I would advise any girl at uni to work in a clothes shop for the discount, even if it's just a Saturday job. One of my mates used to work in TopShop so we got 50 per cent off in there, which was amazing.

Call that a dress?!

My style went a bit mad when I was at university. I'd always been pretty confident with what I wore when I lived at home, but you can't go too crazy when you live with your parents. And I think for that reason I was a bit over-excited because suddenly there were no boundaries. I started wearing tops as dresses so I had my arse hanging out. It saved me loads of money though! The average dress is about £50–£60, but your average top is about £20–£30. I was saving myself 50 per cent . . . but getting very chilly legs in the process.

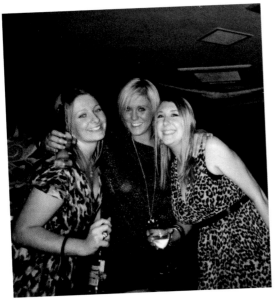

With my Kookai girls, wearing a 'dress' that was most definitely designed to be a top!

I always used to buy my shoes in Shelley's back in the day because it was the first place I ever worked, and it made a real impression on me. I worked with a lot of older girls and they always used to talk to me about quality and even now I spend most money on shoes and bags.

I'm happy to wear a £1 dress if I've got a good pair of shoes in my feet. I'll wear a dress from TopShop or River Island if it suits me, but I'll have Louboutins and a Prada handbag with it. I'm not saying that's what everyone should do, but that's what works for me. I believe accessories make an outfit and they can elevate something that's inexpensive.

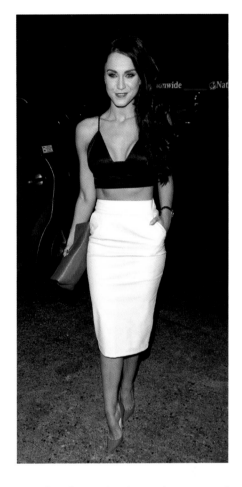

I've got a lovely red Mulberry clutch and some red Celeb Boutique shoes I went through a phase of wearing a lot. It got to the point where people on Instagram were like 'She's wearing them again!' But so what? They go with every outfit, they're good quality and they last well. Shoes and bags are always worth investing in, but you can be more frugal with clothes.

The main style staples I think you should allow yourself to invest in are a really good pair of black shoes, a lovely everyday bag, a great clutch, a good coat, a really nice pair of sunglasses and a classic little black dress. Those things form the basis of your wardrobe and will last you for ever. Once you have your essentials you can build everything else around them.

> **It got to the point where people on Instagram were like 'She's wearing them again!' But so what?**

A lot of girls at uni would go to lectures in jeans and a baggy jumper and then go straight out on the lash, but I didn't. I was a Geordie and the people I was knocking about with were Scousers. We'd go to uni in onesies and trackies, but the minute we were out on the lash you knew about it.

If we were going out on a weekend we'd start doing our fake tan on a Wednesday and we'd have our eyelashes and extensions ready. Scousers take it even further than Geordies. I knew girls who would get their hair blow-dried every time they went out, or they'd get their make-up professionally done to go out on a Thursday. It almost made me step things up a gear because I wanted to keep up with what they were doing.

I'd happily go to the pub for lunch with the lads in a hoodie, but as soon as the evening came I'd go home and take three hours to get ready. I wore a lot of underwear as outerwear back then – basques tucked into skirts and little bra tops with trousers.

Even now if you catch me on a night out and I'm not dressed up it's because the night has been a spur of the moment thing.

It usually means I've had a couple of drinks with my lunch and I haven't stopped. That's the only time you'll see me on a night out in jeans.

I had two looks at uni: full-on glamour or homeless. There was no in between for me, and I'm still the same now. If I'm working on a book I'm in a tracksuit with my hair piled on top of my head and no make-up. But if I'm going out, my hair and make-up has taken a good amount of time.

If I know I'm going to get papped on a night out the glamour has to be full watt. But on the days I don't have to dress up, why would I? I know I've got that polished side of me in my locker and I'm not insecure about looking scruffy, so on the days when I don't have to bother, I don't bother!

Make-up fails

I was never great at doing my own make-up. I could just about do it at uni but I look back at pictures and it wasn't great. I tried to make an effort and I wore eyelashes and things but I didn't look the best. I just wanted to be *very* brown with lashings of mascara and MAC Lipglass, which used to leak all over my bag. Lads probably hated it but I thought it made me look so sexy. It was only other girls who liked lip gloss, and we even used to use it on our eyes because we thought it made them look a bit dewy. It actually just looked greasy and I used to get my eyelashes stuck in it.

Eyebrows have only become a big thing in the last few years and I didn't even own an eyebrow pencil back then, so essentially I looked a bit like a boiled egg. I don't think I had my eyebrows waxed until I was 19 or 20, and now I'm glad I didn't because big eyebrows are a *thing*.

I used to buy my eyelashes for a fiver a pair and I'd recycle them until they looked like spiders. They'd last me for about two weeks and would look horrific at times, but I couldn't afford to keep replacing them.

I've only really got into make-up in the last few years when I started getting my make-up done professionally for shoots. Now I'm aware that you need things like a primer. If you'd mentioned a primer to me ten years ago I'd have thought you were painting your house. I ask make-up artists as they're working on my face what they're doing, but I'm not artistic so I find it hard to replicate anything. That's not to say I *can't* and I have built up my own make-up bag now, but I do love it when make-up artists do it for me.

I used to be obsessed with Maybelline Dream Matte Mousse when I was younger. It came in a tiny little pot and it was like Angel Delight for your face. I'd use the darkest one you could get and put it all over my face and neck. I certainly didn't know about contouring back then, and I didn't know how to use eyeshadow so I didn't wear it.

My going-out beauty routine would be as follows: I'd put on my mousse, powder over the top, then put tons of black mascara and some lashes on. Then I'd finish it off with lip gloss and put my blonde hair extensions in, which I'd buy from a shop next to the precinct in Liverpool. I'd buy these awful clip-ins and there weren't enough for how thick my hair was at the top so you could totally tell I had them in. I was a holy show but I loved it and I thought I looked great. To be fair, most of the time I was so pissed half an hour after I went out I didn't care what I looked like anyway. You didn't have phones with cameras back then, or Twitter or Instagram, so there was no danger of someone taking a dodgy photo of you unless they'd brought their camera with them. And even then, the picture quality was so bad you could get away with beauty murder.

My golden fashion rules

✳ Get the size that fits you. It sounds really obvious but people don't always do it. Remember that no one can see the label inside your dress, but they can see how it looks on the outside. No one knows if you're wearing a size 6 or a size 16, but it's really obvious if you're wearing a dress that is too tight. This infamous photo of me in a yellow dress is a prime example. How it fits is what's important. Clothes that are too small make you look bigger.

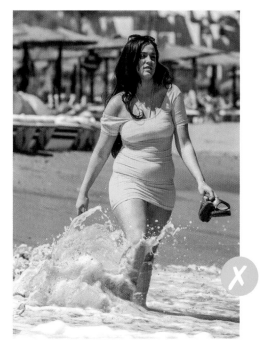

✳ Equally, buying clothes that are way too big isn't flattering because you can swamp yourself. We all have those days where we feel bloated and rubbish and we want to wear a massive jumper to cover ourselves up, but all you'll do is make yourself look bigger. Buy things that fit you well and have that go-to pair of jeans or leather trousers and an oversized white shirt if you're having an off day. That look is so classy and it can hide a multitude of sins. Don't hide away and drown yourself in ill-fitting garments.

✳ Don't speed or panic shop. Changing rooms are frightening and I hate everything about them. I hate the lighting, I hate the fact they're always boiling and I hate the fact you always feel rushed. But *not* trying stuff on is the biggest mistake people make. As awful as they are, take your time in the changing rooms. Or buy clothes online so you can try things on in the comfort of your bedroom.

✳ Take things back! I'm bad for ordering things online in a rush and then when they arrive they're a little bit too snug and I think I'll lose weight and slim into them. Instead they just sit in my wardrobe with the label still on making me feel guilty until I get rid of them. If it's cost me a lot of money I'll probably wear it once and feel really uncomfortable because I'm spilling out of it or you can see my knickers through it, but I'll feel like I *should* because it's expensive. If something isn't right, return it.

✳ Don't ever think 'This will do', 'I'll slim into it' or 'I'll get it just in case'. You should love *everything* you buy. Even while you're sweating your tits off and stressed to death in a changing room, you should still think something looks good before you buy it. If you're feeling indecisive, go shopping with a friend who will be totally honest with you.

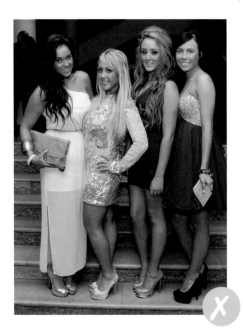

✳ Stick to what suits you. Don't think that just because something looks good on your mate or a model it's going to look good on you. Find your style and stick to it. I hate this picture because you can see how uncomfortable I am in what I'm wearing. It's easy to get overwhelmed in a situation and wear what you *think* you should wear rather than what you *want* to wear. Here I've got too many accessories on and the bag is totally the wrong colour. I didn't own a gold one at the time so I whacked on a bangle in the same colour as the bag to try and tie it in and it doesn't work.

✳ Buy back-ups. Once you find a style or outfit that suits you don't be afraid to get it in several different colours – you'll spot a version of this dress I wore on *Loose Women* elsewhere in the book! Or if you really love it, get another one exactly the same if you know you're going to wear it to death. If you discover something that really suits your body shape, buy two. Half the battle of shopping is finding something you love, so if you find a great LBD or a jumpsuit that can be an ongoing staple, stock up.

✳ More is more. This lace 'dress' is a classic example of me thinking that because I've lost weight I can wear anything I like. This look is not sexy and you don't have to show everything in order to get attention.

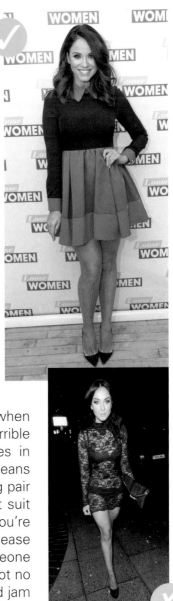

✳ Jeans must be the bane of every woman's life but we all need them. Every store has a slightly different size and fit, especially now that women's jeans seem to have tiny waists and ridiculously long legs. Unfortunately there's no getting out of it: you have to try them on. I tend to go up a size in jeans. So if you're a size 8, buy a size 10. There's nothing worse than people having muffin tops or double bumming, when the denim cuts right into their cheeks. It's also horrible when people get really overly tight jeans with holes in so their flesh pokes through. There's just no need. Jeans should be comfortable, and if you've got a good-fitting pair they can take you anywhere. Don't panic if you don't suit skinnies. Flares are coming back and they're great if you're pear shaped. Dark denim is also super flattering, but please get the length right. There's nothing worse than someone wearing massively long jeans so it looks like they've got no feet. Or ones that are too short so you want to spread jam on their shoes and invite the jeans down for a picnic.

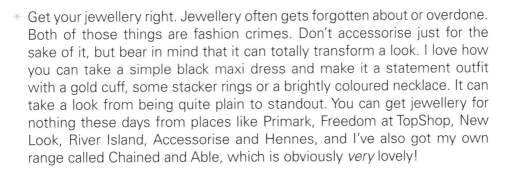

✳ Get your jewellery right. Jewellery often gets forgotten about or overdone. Both of those things are fashion crimes. Don't accessorise just for the sake of it, but bear in mind that it can totally transform a look. I love how you can take a simple black maxi dress and make it a statement outfit with a gold cuff, some stacker rings or a brightly coloured necklace. It can take a look from being quite plain to standout. You can get jewellery for nothing these days from places like Primark, Freedom at TopShop, New Look, River Island, Accessorise and Hennes, and I've also got my own range called Chained and Able, which is obviously *very* lovely!

How I fought the Fresher's 15 . . . and won!

As I've mentioned, I was fresh back from Magaluf when I went to uni and all I'd been doing was working, drinking and sleeping. I'd work all night and then at 6 a.m. I'd go to a place Le Café with all the people I worked with. It was basically an all-day rave disguised as a café that sold drinks called Game Changers, Headf*cks and Amputated Legs (because you couldn't walk after you'd had one).

We'd get wrecked, have a cheese toastie and go to bed until around 4 p.m. Then I'd wake up, go down to the beach, have a bit of dinner and go to work again, so I wasn't eating much and I was walking everywhere. So when I arrived at uni I was slim and brown, but it didn't take me long to bugger that up.

The first year of uni is all about having a good time and I could do whatever I wanted. That independence was lethal so I was having Haribos for breakfast and tons of carbs for my other meals. There was a Subway across the road from me, the Student Union sold great burgers, a place called Hannah's Bar did amazing curly fries, and a shop down the road called The Ten to Ten sold delicious flapjacks. I knew so little about nutrition at the time I genuinely thought flapjacks were healthy. I didn't realise that the oats and raisins were bound together with sugar and butter.

I'd have massive nights out drinking cheap vodka and Red Bull, and then I'd stumble home and eat chips and kebabs. I remember going back to Newcastle for Christmas in my first year and trying on the clothes I'd left behind. None of them fitted and I was gutted.

My friends were really shocked when they saw me. I'd always been a curvy 10 and I went up to a large 12 or a small 14 in three months. That's pretty impressive, but because everyone else at uni was in the same boat and we were all eating terribly, I didn't notice it go on.

I knew I had to do something so when I went back to uni I joined a gym that was right across the road from my halls. It did a really cheap student rate and it was about a two-minute walk so I had no excuse not to go. Some of my friends joined too, which made it easier. A gym buddy is always good.

I started going regularly and I met loads more people there. Some of the personal trainers were also bouncers on the doors of clubs so I killed two birds with one stone. Not only was I getting fit and meeting hot Scouse blokes, I was also jumping the queues when I went out. It was another way for me to spread my wings.

The gym helped me fight the dreaded Fresher's 15 and it made me feel much more confident. I would definitely recommend joining a gym at uni if you can afford it. But I also want to say *chill out* if you put on a bit of weight when you first move out of home. Everyone does, and it'll come off in the end. Uni is the only place you come back after Christmas slimmer than you were before.

Moving out of halls and into a house with friends in my second year made things easier as well because we cooked together and ate more healthily. I was also happier, and I didn't want to put the weight back on. I became more aware of what I was putting in my mouth, and that helped to keep the weight off.

How to stay in shape when all you want to do is eat pizza and go out on the lash

✳ Sleep-deprived people make poorer food choices so stay on track by grabbing a nap or early night after a big night out.

✳ Join a gym near where you live to make it more likely you'll actually *go*.

✳ Plan your workouts around your day. If you come home and know that once you've sat down you won't go out again, take your gym gear and go on the way home from uni instead.

✳ If your hangover is so bad you can't train properly, try just doing 30 minutes on the cross trainer or going for a walk. Drink plenty of water while doing this and you'll feel much better for having made the effort.

✳ Try to stretch for 10–15 minutes after workouts. It will enable your body to recover faster and help you feel less sore.

✳ Get a housemate to go to the gym with you. You'll hold each other accountable on days you don't want to go.

✳ Always have a banana in your gym bag in case you overdo it and start to feel faint. Especially if you're hungover.

✳ You might think doing a few sit-ups will give you a flat stomach, but it's actually training your full body with resistance exercises and HIIT (high-intensity interval training) workouts that'll be most effective at melting that fat. Find out more about HIIT on page 78.

✳ Lacking confidence in the gym? Avoid busy times and start by going mid-mornings or mid-afternoon when it'll be quieter.

✳ Busy gym? You can almost always guarantee that the leg equipment will be free so jump on the leg press or leg curl. Training legs is a brilliant way of burning lots of calories.

✳ Feeling like you aren't making progress? Snap some pictures of yourself in front of the mirror and take some tape measurements. Repeat these every two weeks because you might be making more progress than you realise.

✳ Writing down what you did in the gym is a great way of making sure you keep progressing. Try tracking your weights and reps. (There are also apps that can help you do this.)

✳ Warm up before you train, even if it's just five minutes of cardio.

✳ Never start with a heavy set of weights. Always build up with plenty of warm-up sets, using lighter weights to build up to your first rep at the full weight.

✳ Feel lost in the gym? Try a class and let the instructor keep you on track.

✳ Plan your sessions around your nights out. If you always go out on a Wednesday, don't expect to be able to train hard on a Thursday.

✳ Got writers' block with that essay? Breaking up your day by blasting out a workout can be a great way of energising yourself and being more productive.

✳ Running can be great for exercise and stress relief but make sure your trainers are right for you. A decent running shop will be able to advise you. Paying for a good pair is far cheaper than costly physio bills for injured knees or ankles.

Spicy chicken tacos with corn salsa

Knowing how to cook one or two filling and nutritious meals for yourself (beans on toast doesn't count) will really help you to stay healthy – and stop your mum worrying!

Ingredients

500g sliced chicken breasts

30g fajita spice mix

3 tablespoons olive oil

8 taco shells

½ large red pepper, seeds removed and cut into long strips

2 onions, sliced

2 garlic cloves, chopped

Guacamole and salad, to serve

Corn salsa

340g can sweetcorn, drained

½ large red pepper, finely chopped

5 spring onions, finely chopped

1 medium-hot red chilli, seeds removed and finely chopped

Juice of 1 lime

Splash of olive oil

Salt and pepper

Method

1. Put the chicken in a bowl and pour over the spice mix and 1 tablespoon of the oil. Turn the chicken until it is coated in the spices. If you have time, cover the bowl containing the chicken with cling film. Leave the chicken to marinate for at least 30 minutes in the fridge, but if there's no time, no problem.

2. Mix together all the ingredients for the corn salsa in a serving bowl and set aside.

3. Preheat the oven to 180° C. Stand the taco shells upright on a baking tray and warm through for 5 minutes.

4. While the tacos are warming up, heat the rest of the oil in a large frying pan over a medium-high heat. Add the chicken, red pepper and onions and stir-fry for 5 minutes or until the chicken is cooked through. Stir in the garlic and a little water and heat through.

5. To serve, spoon the spicy chicken, peppers and onions into the taco shells and top with a good spoonful of the corn salsa. Serve with guacamole and salad. (You can use the guacamole recipe from page 94, if you want something healthier than the shop-bought variety.)

WORK IT

Hustle your way to the top in style.

4

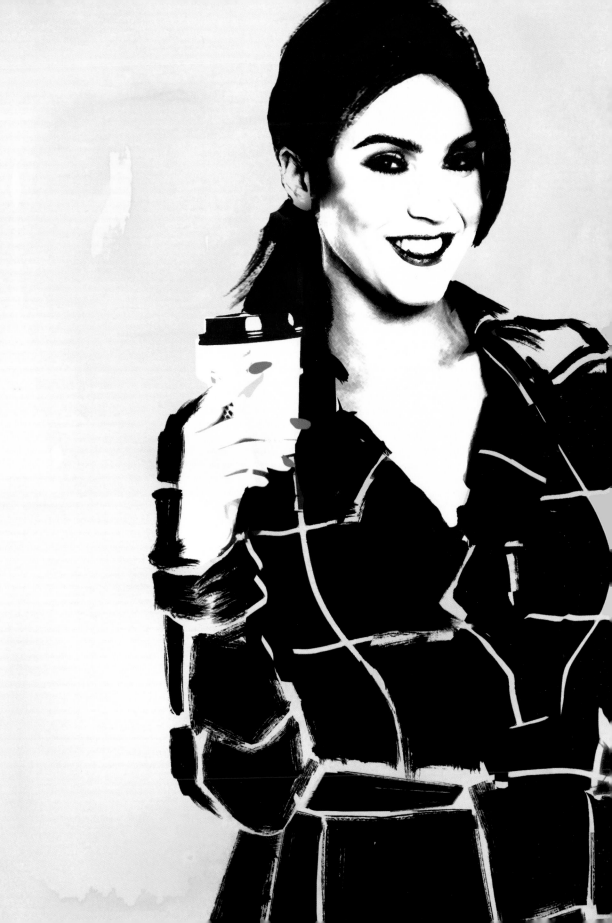

How I got turned down for a job at Aldi

Starting full-time work is always a bit daunting because you're starting another big phase of your life and you feel like so much is going to change.

I thought life after uni would be like it is in American films. I honestly thought I'd throw my cap in the air and then some high-flying businessman would appear from nowhere and offer me an amazing job. But sadly it's just not like that.

The year I left university, 200,000 students graduated and there were 20,000 jobs available. I was in trouble, especially as my degree wasn't very specialised or geared to a certain profession like sports science or law. I did drama and media and cultural studies, so what did that make me qualified for? I was floundering.

I moved back home, thinking it was temporary and that I'd be heading to Manchester or London in no time to kick off my incredible career. At that time I thought I wanted to be a journalist – but I kept changing my mind all the time. Uni hadn't made things any clearer for me on the work front.

I'd never really known what I wanted to do. Friends of mine wanted to be teachers or solicitors, so they all chose courses that were very specific and would give them the skills they needed. All I knew was that I didn't want any kind of predictability in my career. I didn't want to have to go to the same office every day and see the same people. Whatever I did, I wanted it to be fast-paced and exciting. (As a side note, I'd just like to say my life is exactly that now.)

The first job I got post-uni was at the clothes shop, G-Star, which was great fun and although it definitely wasn't what I wanted to be doing for the rest of my life, it was nice to take a bit of a step back from things. I'd spent three years at uni thinking about money and making sure I got my work in on time, so it was nice that I had nothing to worry about because I had the security of my parents again.

I told myself I'd have six months at home and then I'd move to a big city with my friend Kailee, where we'd rent an amazing studio apartment and live the high life, working glamorous fast-paced jobs, wearing pencil skirts (which we thought were the height of sophistication at the time) and dating international models. But instead I kept spending all my money on going out. Being at uni had taught me about managing my money, but apparently I forgot everything the minute I stepped back through the door of my family home.

I'd get paid on a Friday and spend £125 on clothes and make-up almost immediately, because I knew that if the worst came to the worst my mam would drive me to work and there was always food in the house. My friends and I would go out on a Friday and roll in on a Sunday and I absolutely loved it. I reverted back to having zero responsibility. So all the great disciplines I'd learnt fell by the wayside, and because my mam had missed me just as much as I'd missed her, I got away with everything.

Although I was being pretty irresponsible, I was still looking for 'proper' jobs. One of the first things I applied for was the management programme at Aldi, because they fast-tracked you on to £40K a year and you got a company car if you were a university graduate. I probably would have hated it but it was such a good package I got lured in by it. I've always wanted to be financially stable and even if I didn't love the idea of the job, the money was good. I didn't actually get the job because I was late to the interview, which is always a bit of a no-no.

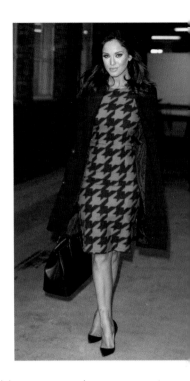

Work is 100 per cent my priority at the moment. The people I hang around with like to play hard, but they work harder. Even if I've had a big night out, I'll still be up the next morning and I'll be wherever I need to be on time with a smile on my face. I am always professional, respectful and nice, even if my head's banging and I'm dreaming of my bed.

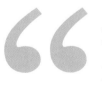

> **Don't moan about not having something; go out and get it. You really can do anything you want to.**

When it comes to your career your vibe attracts your tribe, and if you're positive and hard-working, you'll have those people around you. It's so much easier to be positive and supportive if you're doing well, and if you've got people around you who are the same. If you're always looking at what someone else has got and whinging about them doing better than you rather than striving to be better yourself, you're never going to be happy. I don't want people like that in my life.

For a while I had certain people, who were doing similar things to me, who would come up to me at parties and say things like: 'I really want another TV show, and I really want people to be more interested in me.' I'd look at them and think, *Why are you telling me this? Get up and do something!* You're the master of your own destiny, but a lot of people would rather have something handed to them than actually have to work for it. Don't moan about not having something; go out and get it. You really can do anything you want to.

I have learnt the hard way that it doesn't matter what industry you're in, you'll get a reputation from the minute you start working. Everyone talks and everyone knows each other, so you have to decide early on what you want that reputation to be.

I've made a lot of mistakes getting to where I am now, and I'll never dispute that or act like my past didn't happen. I own it because I've had to apologise for it and make amends.

When I was on *Geordie Shore* and I was having a bad time with my ex, Ricci, I would sometimes take it out on crew members. I wouldn't be as polite and respectful as I normally am and that makes me feel terrible. I was stupid, young, naive and probably a little bit arrogant to think that people would forget it or they wouldn't tell others. But they did.

I'd do some work on another show, and crew members would tell me they 'knew someone' who worked on *Geordie Shore*. I knew they were really saying to me: 'We've got your card marked because we know what you're capable of.'

That was when I started to realise how small most industries are. I wanted to make a career out of TV and I was horrified at how I'd behaved at times. I'd allowed my personal life to affect my professional life, and that is not okay.

Always be the best version of yourself you can be. Put your best foot forward and you can't go far wrong. Apparently when Take That made their big comeback, people were lining up to help them out because they had been so nice to everyone the first time around. They were always polite and remembered people's names, from runners to make-up artists. By the time they gave their career a second shot, those runners had become execs, and they still remembered the time Gary Barlow asked them if they wanted a cup of tea. The saying 'be nice to everyone on the way up because you'll meet them on the way down' is so true and it's a motto that I live by.

I'm a Celebrity had an 800-strong crew, and I endeavoured to remember everyone's name on that show. To make a person feel valued in the workplace – no matter what level you're both on – means the world. Just think how you feel when someone you look up to remembers your name or thanks you for your contribution. It makes you feel amazing, and you should be as kind to others as you want others to be to you.

Try not to be a knob at work. In fact, if you take anything from this book, please always remember not to be a knob in any area of your life.

How to smash your CV

It may seem old-fashioned, but CVs are still considered really important when you're trying to get a job. We got taught how to do a good CV at school and I think it's part of the reason I have never, ever struggled to get a job. I worked in retail from the age of 15 and people were always coming in with CVs looking for work. Sometimes it would be heartbreaking because they'd shuffle in apologetically and not make any eye contact when they handed it in.

It's just as important – if not more important – how you present yourself when you hand that CV over. Look presentable and smile. Fake it till you make it. Even if you're not feeling 100 per cent confident, strap on your lady balls, smile and look your potential employer in the eye. They don't need to know that you're a bag of nerves on the inside.

✳ You don't have to have the most on your CV for it to be a winning one; just make the most of what you've got. People mainly want to know that you're keen, competent, ambitious, raring to go and confident.

✳ Remember that everyone has to start somewhere. Even when I didn't have much paid work experience, I went and helped my mam out with her charity work. I also helped my auntie in her office because she worked in HR, so I learnt workplace skills and how to get on in an office environment. This all showed employers that I had initiative.

✳ Even things like being on your local netball team count. It shows that you can work as part of a team and you've got dedication. They're the kind of things employers will look for. Being a team player is a massive part of working anywhere. No matter how small you think your achievements are, they could be what a company is looking for.

✳ Don't be afraid to big yourself up. No achievement is too small to go on a CV as long as you word it correctly. One of the things I was proudest of was that I was a house captain in middle school, because that showed that my teachers trusted me enough to give me some level of responsibility and leadership. I think 'house captain' is still on my CV now actually.

✳ Ask for help with your CV and get it proofread by someone else, or even a few people. Spelling mistakes are a massive no-no. It looks sloppy and lazy, and no one wants to employ someone like that.

✳ Constantly update it and don't rest on your laurels. The minute you get a job or do something that you consider to be CV worthy, pop it on.

What to do (and what definitely *not* to do) in an interview

✳ Interviews are obviously key to getting a job, but the thing is, within about three seconds of you walking into the room, the person interviewing you has decided whether you're in the running to get the job or not. No matter what comes out of your mouth after those three seconds, you've pretty much already ruled yourself in or out. It's all down to how you present yourself initially – just like on a first date!

✳ Dress for the situation. If you're going for an office job, it's best to go for something quite traditional to begin with. A good suit or trousers and a shirt doesn't have to cost the earth – or make you look forty years older than you are!

✳ You might know someone who works at the company you're applying to and know that they wear jeans to work; that doesn't mean it's okay for you to wear jeans to the interview. You need to show them you mean business and dress for the job you want.

✳ I remember going for an interview at Warehouse wearing clothes that were in line with what they were selling at the time. That showed I'd done my research and I was on-trend. If you're trying to get a job in a clothes shop, things like that go a long way.

✳ If you're going for a job on a make-up counter, make sure your make-up is immaculate. But don't go along to an interview for a job in a library looking like you're going on a night out. You're not misrepresenting yourself, but you do have to be realistic about your look.

✳ The person interviewing you may seem really intimidating but don't let it faze you. I remember being interviewed by a woman who seemed like the scariest person in the world. She was gorgeous, dressed immaculately and seemed the most mature, repsonsible and impressive human I'd ever met. I was petrified of her, but I got the job and a couple of months later we went on a night out and I saw her drunk. She was chatting to me in McDonald's with cheeseburger all over her face and it humanised her. That was the moment I realised she was normal too. So when you're sitting in an interview with someone who seems to have their life completely together, imagine them with their face in a bowl of cheesy chips and remember that they're had a first interview at some point too. They've been you and they're no different.

✳ Interviews only have as much weight and gravity as you give them, so if you chill out the chances are the interview will feel more relaxed as well.

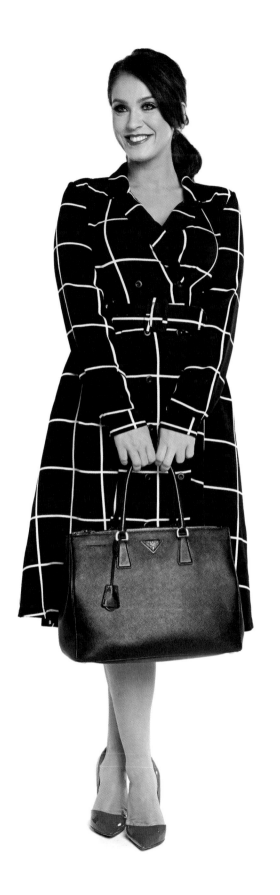

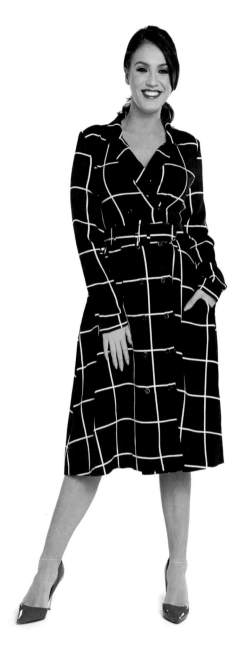

You've got to dress for the job you want.

✳ When you're actually in the interview, do your best to stay calm. Fidgeting isn't ideal. Remember that the interviewer has obviously seen something either in you or on your CV they like, and if you don't actually get the job it's not the end of the world because it's all good practice.

✳ Be positive and sell yourself. The interviewer is looking for you to tell them why they should hire you.

✳ Don't be too hard on yourself if you don't get the job. It doesn't mean that you are completely unemployable! They may have seen someone else who exactly fitted what they were looking for, and there's nothing you can do about that but dust yourself off and try again somewhere else. But you are entitled to feedback so it's worth giving them a call to see if you can pick up some good pointers for improving your interview technique.

✳ There are some great videos on YouTube that will help with interviews, and if you are really nervous, ask a friend to grill you with some sample questions beforehand.

Good things to say in interviews

✓ 'I'm a team-player.'

✓ 'I love the company and I think I've got loads of qualities that would benefit you.'

✓ 'I love learning new things.'

✓ 'I'm good at timekeeping.'

And if you really want the job, tell them! Just before you walk out, say something like, 'I'd love this job' or 'I'd be good at this'. It's such a positive and confident note to end on. I remember after I had my interview for the jungle they asked me if there was anything I'd like to add and I just said, 'I'll smash this!' And look how that ended up.

Things that aren't so good to say:

✗ 'I get bored easily.'

✗ (If it's an interview for a shop) 'Will I get free clothes and/or a discount?'

✗ 'There are a few dates I definitely won't be able to work because I've got things booked in my diary.'

✗ 'I'm not really a people person.'

✗ 'I love getting mortal every weekend.'

How to dress to impress and still look chic

Work outfits should be smart, comfortable and sassy. Remember that you've got to be in it all day, so you don't want to be wearing something you don't feel good in, or something that feels too tight or has horrible itchy material.

Obviously, as with interviews, you need to dress to suit your job. Don't turn up to a stint in a trendy clothes shop wearing a power suit.

The dress on page 69 is a great shape because it's heavily belted and nips you in at the waist. I've got it in plain black as well and it's sexy and understated. This can be worn in any season with any colour, which gives you a lot of shoe options.

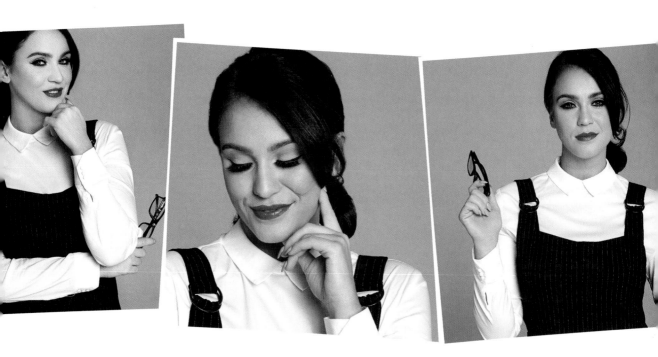

Everyone should have a good, crisp white shirt in their wardrobe. It's a capsule item and goes with so many things. Own a couple if you can. Just by undoing a couple of buttons you can take your work outfit from day to night. You can morph from 'office worker of the month' to the girl who gets free drinks in the bar. I love a pinafore too, because it looks both smart and cute. You can throw a cool jacket or coat over the top and look really businessy, or classic and chic once you take it off.

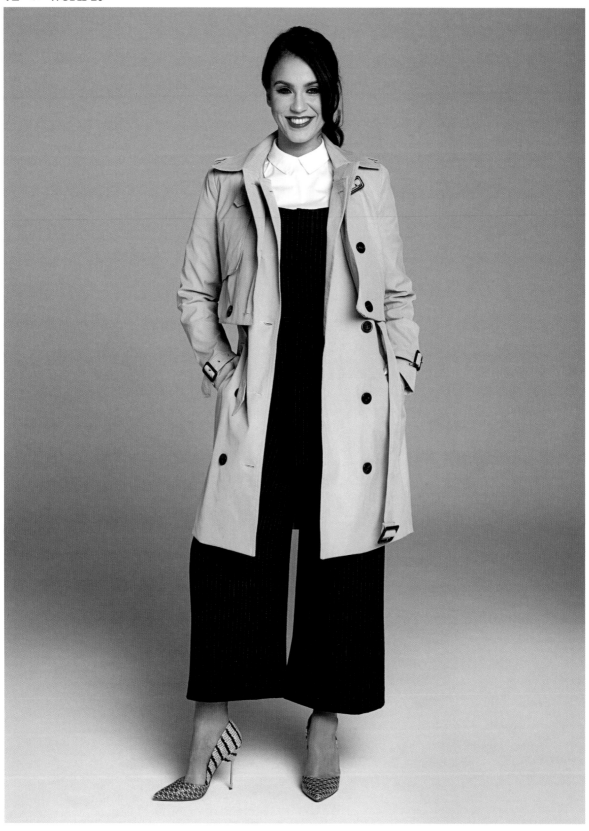

My favourite working hairstyle. Looks chic, says you mean business

✳ Hair needs to be blow-dried nice and sleek for this look, but you can keep a curl in the ends if you want a nice bouncy ponytail. You can also tong it if you want extra curl.

✳ Separate out your fringe and set it in a pin curl so it's out of the way.

✳ Backcomb the whole of the top section of the hair to create height. Most people just backcomb the root, but you should go right from the root all the way to the ends of the hair.

✳ Completely smooth down the underneath of the hair so it's nice and sleek, and then lightly brush the backcombed section over the top and smooth it down.

✳ Brush out your fringe and secure it behind your ears. If you've got a long fringe you can blend the ends in with the rest of your hair.

✳ Secure your hair in place using a bobble, and then take a piece of hair from the ponytail and wrap it around it so it hides the bobble. Either tuck it into the bobble or secure underneath with a pin so it can't be seen.

✳ Use a tail comb to get the height you want on your backcombed bump. I like mine quite chic and sleek; just high enough to have a bit of a Bardot going on.

✳ Spray with Elnett hairspray and you're good to go.

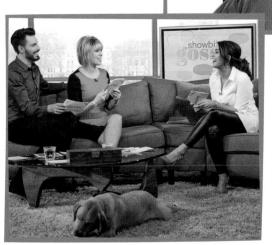

White shirt + leather trousers = sassy work outfit nailed!

My worst jobs ever

I once had a job in a bar in Newcastle called Sam Jacks, which was cowboy-themed and required me to wear nothing other than a bikini and a pair of leather chaps. It wasn't ideal in the winter, and we used to get loads of loud, randy stag dos coming in making leery comments. I didn't last very long.

I also worked in a restaurant called Savanna's in Ibiza. I was under the impression I was going to be a hostess and I thought I'd be floating around in a maxi dress looking serene and enticing people in. In reality they expected me to wait on tables and run around with those fancy two-foot plates that had about three prawns on them. All the Spanish employees had been working there for years and were experts at balancing five plates on their little fingers, and they used to mutter under their breath at me as I struggled with one. I felt so useless and just wanted to be getting drunk with all my mates.

I think my worst job though was when I worked in a broadband call centre. That was hell on earth. I am not good with authority and I hate following rules. It was one of those places where creativity was not encouraged and it went against everything I enjoy. I was always getting into trouble for wearing the wrong thing even though I only spoke to people over the phone. I'd also get told off for being late a lot, or not reading out the five golden broadband rules. I'd constantly pretend I needed the toilet so I'd be put to the back of the queue for calls. It was the worst and I still don't know the five golden broadband rules.

Please don't ever make me go back there.

A healthy work lunch that's easy, virtuous and bloody delicious

Staying healthy while you're working can be a nightmare. I'm always on the go and it can feel so much easier to grab some fast food while I'm rushing around between appointments than to sit down and take the time to eat something healthy. And I've spent enough time in offices to know that there's always someone's birthday cake or sweets they've brought back from Tenerife to tempt you.

I know from experience that stuffing yourself with empty calories might feel good at the time, but it'll lead to massive energy slumps and play havoc with your weight. You'll feel so much better – and enjoy your lunch so much more – if you can find the time to prepare something like this chicken and roast vegetable salad the night before.

Chicken, quinoa and roasted vegetables *(serves 1)*

Ingredients

1 carrot

1 courgette

1 red pepper

1 tablespoon olive oil

¼ cup quinoa (rinsed)

1 chicken breast

A dash of balsamic
   vinegar

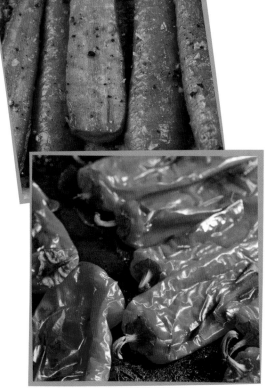

Method

1. Preheat the oven to 200° C.

2. Chop the vegetables into thick (approx 2cm) chunks and drizzle with the olive oil.

3. Spread the vegetables thinly over a large baking tray and roast for 30–35 minutes, stirring once during cooking.

4. Meanwhile, preheat the grill, then grill the chicken until cooked through. Once cooled slice into bite-sized chunks. (To check if chicken is cooked properly, pierce with a knife. If the juices run clear, you're good to go. If they're pink or you're in doubt, whack it back in for a bit longer.)

5. Place the quinoa in a small saucepan and cover with ½ cup of boiling water. Bring to the boil, then cover and reduce to a simmer for 10–12 minutes until the water has been absorbed.

6. Once the vegetables have been roasted, mix them with the chicken chunks and quinoa. Allow to cool and then refrigerate.

7. Transfer to a suitable container and add a dash of balsamic vinegar before taking to work.

Benefits: *Quinoa is a gluten-free superfood that is packed with nutrients – especially minerals – and is a good source of fibre, so it's a brilliant all-rounder. And roasting carrot and red pepper in a little oil increases the amount of the antioxidant beta-carotene that your body can absorb.*

Healthy on-the-go snacks that will stop you grabbing crisps

Pre-preparing a snack like this seed mix and carrying it in your bag, or keeping it in a container in your desk drawer, will really help you to avoid snacking on crisps or other salt-and/or sugar-heavy snacks.

Toasted seed and cashew mix

Ingredients

1/3 cup cashew nuts

1/3 cup sunflower seeds

1/3 cup pumpkin seeds

1 tablespoon tahini (puréed sesame seeds)

1 tablespoon tamari soy sauce

1 tablespoon olive oil

1 teaspoon frozen chopped red chilli

Method

1. Preheat the oven to 150° C and line a large baking tray with greaseproof paper.

2. Mix the cashew nuts and seeds in a bowl.

3. Mix the wet ingredients and chilli together, then pour them into the bowl of seeds and stir well.

4. Spread the mix thinly onto the lined baking tray and place in the oven for 15–20 minutes, stirring once or twice.

5. Once you remove the tray from the oven, allow the nut and seed mix to cool and then transfer into an airtight container.

6. Take a small handful with you as a snack, in a small container or freezer bag.

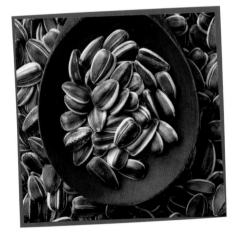

Benefits: *Seeds and cashew nuts are a great source of protein and healthy fats, meaning that they can help keep you feeling full until your next meal time. Pumpkin and sunflower seeds are rich in skin-healthy zinc and essential fatty acids, which will both help to give you a glow. Nuts and seeds are packed with minerals and other nutrients needed for energy production to keep you going for longer.*

Apple and almond oat bites

Sometimes you do need something a bit sweet to snack on in the afternoon, to get you through that 3 o'clock slump. These oaty treats are a fantastic biscuit substitute, and perfect with a cup of green tea.

Ingredients

2 cups whole oats

½ cup ground almonds

2 tablespoons ground flax seeds

1 large pinch of sea salt

¼ cup almond butter

3 tablespoons honey

¼ cup almond milk

¼ cup unsweetened apple sauce

1 teaspoon vanilla extract

Coconut oil

Method

1. Preheat the oven to 180° C and grease a 20cm x 20cm baking tin with coconut oil.

2. In a large mixing bowl, combine the dry ingredients.

3. In a medium bowl whisk or blend the wet ingredients together, then add to the dry ingredients and mix thoroughly.

4. Transfer the mix into the tin and bake for 20 minutes until golden brown on top.

5. Allow to cool slightly and then turn the content of the tin out onto a chopping board.

6. Once cooled, cut the oat bake into small squares. These can be refrigerated for a few days or frozen in small batches. When you're ready to head out, take a few out the freezer, and they'll be ready by the time a snack attack hits!

Can't find unsweetened apple sauce in a health food shop? Try organic baby food instead for pure puréed fruit with no added sugar.

Benefits: *Oats are a great source of slow-release energy, and combined with the protein and healthy fats in almonds this snack will help curb any hunger cravings. And as well as giving you healthy fats, almonds are packed with minerals such as calcium for healthy bones and magnesium for energy production.*

Exercises you can fit around work, so there's no excuse!

For people with a busy schedule, it's about doing the best you can in a short period of time. This is where high-intensity workouts are ideal.

This means working your full body with high-tempo, high-intensity routines. Think sprinter rather than a marathon runner – we're going flat-out for a short period of time.

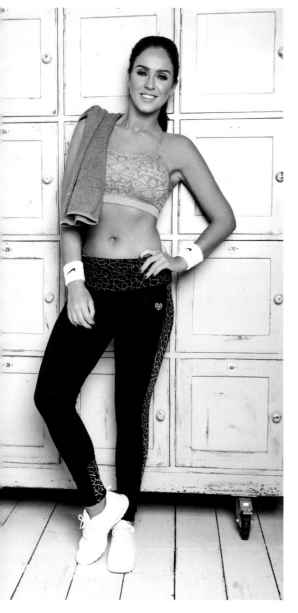

A great way of doing this is with an 'every minute, on the minute' workout. This involves setting the stopwatch on your phone in front of you – every minute you will do a set exercise for a certain amount of reps (for example 20 burpees) then you'll rest for the remainder of the minute. If it takes you 40 seconds, you get 20 seconds, rest. Once that timer gets to the start of the next minute, you'll start your next exercise.

You could do this for 15–20 minutes – it's a great way of cramming a lot of work into a short period of time. And as you can see you don't need a lot of room: this could easily be done in a hotel room, your bedroom or even your office!

Here's a sample workout:

Bodyweight Squats: 20

Stand with your feet shoulder-width apart, bend your knees and push your hips back as if you were sitting down. Lower until your thighs are parallel with the floor and, pushing through your heels, come back up. You can actually sit onto a chair or bench if you are struggling with this.

Push Ups: 20

These are great for your chest, shoulders and arms. Place your hands on the floor, shoulder-width apart, directly under your shoulders. Either lift up onto your toes or your knees – this is your start position with your arms straight. From here bend your elbows and imagine squeezing your shoulder blades together as you lower, pause just shy of the floor and push back up.

Burpees: 20

These are tough! Get in position as if you were doing a push up, from here bend your legs and jump them forwards so your knees are in line with your hands, then stand up and jump in the air. Place your hands back on the floor, jump your feet back to the start position. That's one burpee.

V-up Crunches: 20

Lie on your back with your arms straight overhead and legs straight. Lift your legs and arms off the floor and bring them together in the air above your hips. If this is too tough, you can bend your legs!

Bodyweight Lunges: 20

Standing with your feet shoulder-width apart, step forwards with one leg and slowly lower your other leg towards the floor, push through your front leg back to the start position then do the same with your other leg.

Repeat for 20 minutes

If you're struggling to get enough rest between exercises reduce them to 15 reps.

And don't underestimate the impact that just being more active can have on your fitness:

✳ Get off the bus a stop earlier and walk the rest of the way to the office

✳ Take the stairs rather than the lift

✳ Take the dog a little further on his walk (if you have one, obviously!)

✳ Get out for a short walk on your lunch break

✳ Rather than catching up with a friend over coffee, why not go for a walk together?

HERE COME THE GIRLS

Everything you need for a perfect girls' night out . . . or in.

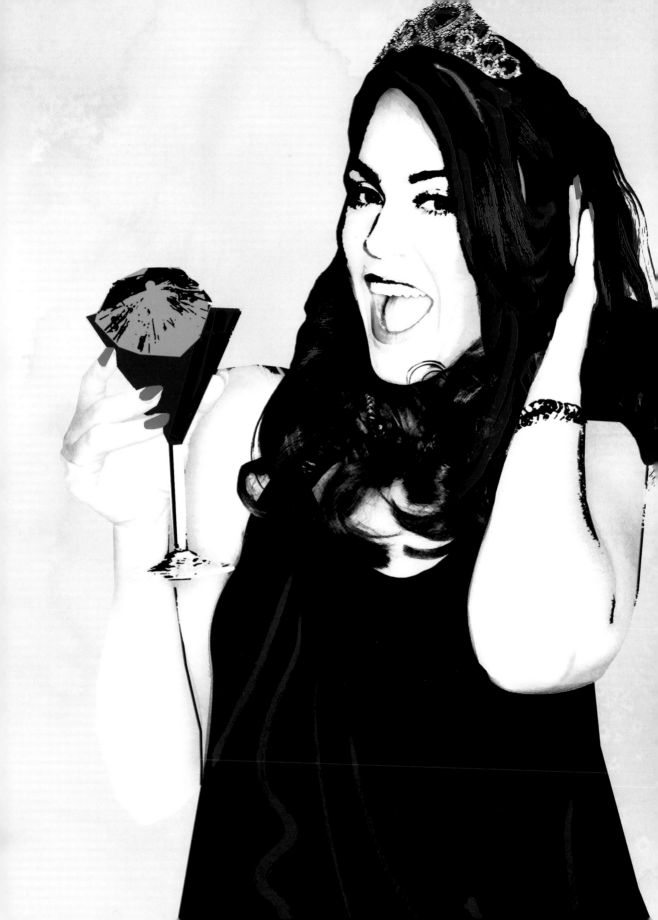

Why getting ready can be the best part of a girls' night out

Always get ready for a girls' night out *with your girls*. Never do it on your own – it's just not as much fun and you want to set yourself up for a great night. I like the house to be full of noise with half-naked women running around asking each other for help doing up their dresses or putting their make-up on.

Half of the going-out process requires a buddy. If you're getting ready on your own, who's going to fake tan your back? Boyfriends are no good for that sort of thing. I once had a friend who used to pay her brother 50p to do it and I remember thinking he'd make someone a good husband one day.

One of my friends is dead good at putting my hair in rollers, and I'll do her eyelashes in return. I'll lend someone my clothes and they'll fake tan my back to say thank you. That's what it's all about, isn't it?

It's so much fun when you're all trying on outfits and you can advise each other and be like 'Your legs look great in that one' or 'That one makes your boobs look amazing'. You want your mates to look and feel the best they possibly can.

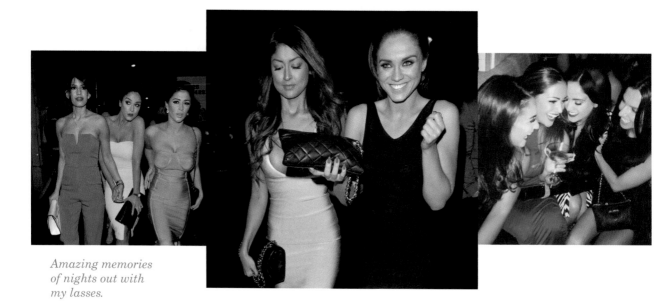

Amazing memories of nights out with my lasses.

Sometimes getting ready is the best part of the night. You're not queuing for the toilet and getting jostled about and there's no wait for your drinks. You're sitting together drinking Prosecco and having a laugh. You can choose the music and have some snacks. But not too many, because as we all know, eating's cheating! Some nibbles are fine, but you want to save the proper eating for when you're out or after you've been drinking. I'll lay on something light like carrot sticks and hummus and crisps and nuts, but you don't want to settle down to masses of scran before you've even got out the door.

Music wise, I like stuff that's about empowering females, so anything by Beyoncé, Little Mix or Cheryl is a winner. You want a playlist that will get you all fired up before you go out.

A girls' night out has to be planned with military precision and you need a captain. I'll make myself the captain, but as I'm not that great when it comes to time-keeping one of my mates will slyly take over that role without me even realising.

I'm the friend who has everyone round to mine, but I'm also the girl who is *always* ready last. Someone else will be in charge of booking the taxi and they'll always tell me it's coming half an hour earlier than it is, so I'm not running around flapping while everyone is shouting at me. A taxi buffer is a really good thing. It's all about teamwork!

Getting-ready playlist

- ☛ *Call My Name* by Cheryl Cole
- ☛ *Black Magic* by Little Mix
- ☛ *Hands to Myself* by Selena Gomez
- ☛ *Stronger* by Britney Spears
- ☛ *Maneater* by Nelly Furtado
- ☛ *Gold Digger* by Kanye West
- ☛ *Bootylicious* by Destiny's Child
- ☛ *Jenny From the Block* by Jennifer Lopez
- ☛ *Run the World (Girls)* by Beyoncé
- ☛ *Spinning Around* by Kylie Minogue
- ☛ *Respect* by Aretha Franklin
- ☛ *Dirrty* by Christina Aguilera
- ☛ *7 Days* by Craig David
- ☛ *You Make Me Wanna* by Usher
- ☛ *Post to Be* by Omarion featuring Chris Brown and Jhene Aiko

That getting-ready time is when we all get to properly catch up. Anything and everything gets discussed and that's how it should be. Once you're out, the chat becomes more superficial and it's more about what you're drinking and who else is in the bar. You're too busy doing shots and dancing to have a proper conversation.

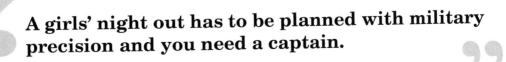

A girls' night out has to be planned with military precision and you need a captain.

What to wear, and how to make sure you're not wearing the same thing as your mate

When we've got a big night coming up, my friends and I start discussing what we're wearing in our WhatsApp group for days, or maybe even weeks, beforehand. We'll discuss what kind of look we're going for and whether it's 'dress casual' or 'full-on glamour', and we'll even send pictures to each other. It builds up the excitement.

My mates and I have all got different styles and different body types, so there's rarely any danger of us wearing the same outfit. And thanks to the WhatsApp group you can be pretty certain that's not going to happen. If you are getting ready at someone else's house, maybe take a couple of options just in case, because someone might go rogue and change their minds at the last minute and you could end up wearing similar things.

There have been times when our group ends up looking like a girlband; in spite of all our efforts not to wear the same thing, we all end up wearing shades of the same colour. I think that's a true testament to how close we are. When that happens you know you're off to a good start and you're going to have a great night. When you walk out of the house and do that last mirror check and think *I look sick and my squad look sick. Watch out men!* It's the best feeling.

When I'm on a girls' night, what I wear isn't necessarily about being sexy; it's more about feeling glamorous and slinky. I'll wear something bodycon with a bit of cleavage showing, or a backless dress. You know all the other girls will be bringing their A-game and I think women try to impress other women far more than they try to impress men. No one has seventeen nude MAC lipsticks for a lad's benefit. They don't even notice them. We all like to get other women's approval and that's a part of the reason we make sure we look amazing.

Shoe game

Personally, when it comes to shoes I wouldn't be seen dead in anything less than a three-inch heel on a night out. Having said that, it doesn't matter what shoes you wear, whether it's kitten heels, ballet pumps or platforms, they have to be comfortable. Girls' nights out are about having fun and dancing all night long and there's nothing worse than a night being brought to a close because a mate is moaning about her feet hurting.

You will never catch me walking out of a club with my shoes in my hand because I make sure I can last the entire night in whatever footwear I choose to put on. I always make sure I take Compede Blister Plasters and Scholl Party Feet, just in case my shoes do start to hurt for any reason. I pop them

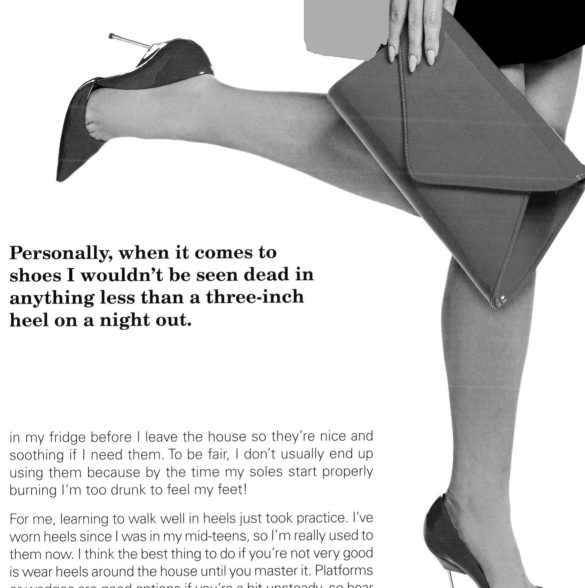

Personally, when it comes to shoes I wouldn't be seen dead in anything less than a three-inch heel on a night out.

in my fridge before I leave the house so they're nice and soothing if I need them. To be fair, I don't usually end up using them because by the time my soles start properly burning I'm too drunk to feel my feet!

For me, learning to walk well in heels just took practice. I've worn heels since I was in my mid-teens, so I'm really used to them now. I think the best thing to do if you're not very good is wear heels around the house until you master it. Platforms or wedges are good options if you're a bit unsteady, so bear that in mind. The thinner the heel the harder shoes are to walk in, so maybe work up to really killer heels.

It may sound like an obvious thing to say but it's a major help if your shoes fit properly. If they're too small when you try them on in a shop, even if they are your usual size, get the next size up and put an insole inside them.

If you do have a particularly tight pair of shoes, pack wet, scrunched-up newspaper tightly inside the front of them and as it dries it will expand and stretch your shoes. Or if you're worried about putting wet newspaper in your new shoes, find a friend with a bigger pair of feet than you and ask them if they'll wear them in for you. I've also got mates who have paid their little brothers to wear their shoes in for them, which is a genius idea.

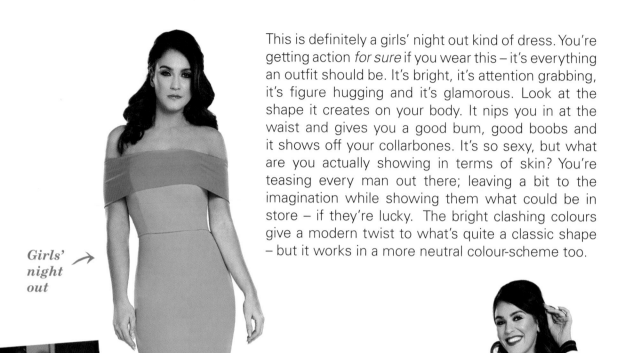

This is definitely a girls' night out kind of dress. You're getting action *for sure* if you wear this – it's everything an outfit should be. It's bright, it's attention grabbing, it's figure hugging and it's glamorous. Look at the shape it creates on your body. It nips you in at the waist and gives you a good bum, good boobs and it shows off your collarbones. It's so sexy, but what are you actually showing in terms of skin? You're teasing every man out there; leaving a bit to the imagination while showing them what could be in store – if they're lucky. The bright clashing colours give a modern twist to what's quite a classic shape – but it works in a more neutral colour-scheme too.

*Girls'
night
out* →

→ *Weeknight
cocktails*

I'd wear this for evening cocktails with the girls on a Thursday. It's not a Saturday outfit, but if you're meeting after work, you've had an hour or so to get ready and you want something cute but casual, this is a winner. It doesn't scream 'I've tried dead hard' and you can feel comfortable in it. It's fun and flirty and I love the fifties, nautical vibe.

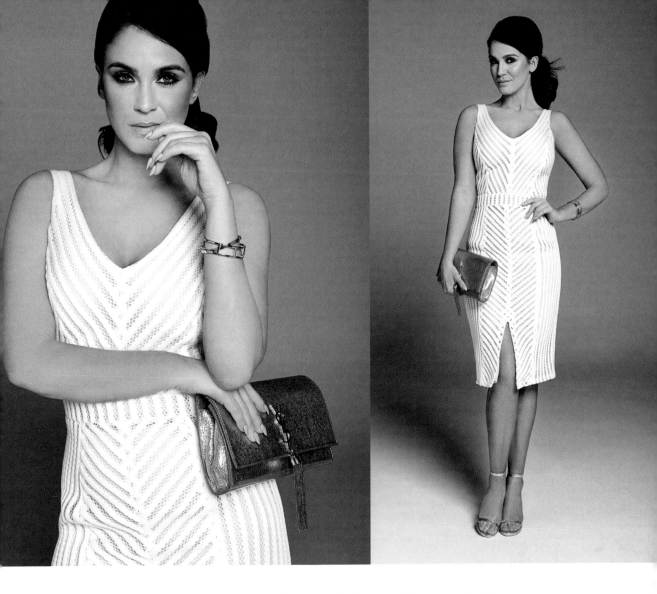

I think white is so classic, timeless and elegant. If you walk into a room wearing white, everyone is going to stare. I know people rave about winter white, but for me white will always signify the start of summer because it looks great with a tan. I know you can fake tan really easily, but it's inevitable that you're going to get it all over your nice pristine outfit, so you're much better off waiting until you have a real tan to wear something like this. A glowing tan, a stunning white dress and gold accessories is an amazing look for a special night out with the girls.

The only downside to wearing white is that you have to be *so* careful. If you're anything like me and you're going out on a night out to let your hair down, you need to face the fact you're going to come back looking a bit manky. If you're going to be brave enough to wear white on a night out, and I salute anyone who does, just be aware that that outfit is not coming home *white*. You seem to attract more stains and I will generally finish the evening looking like I've rolled around on the floor. Maybe steer clear of red wine!

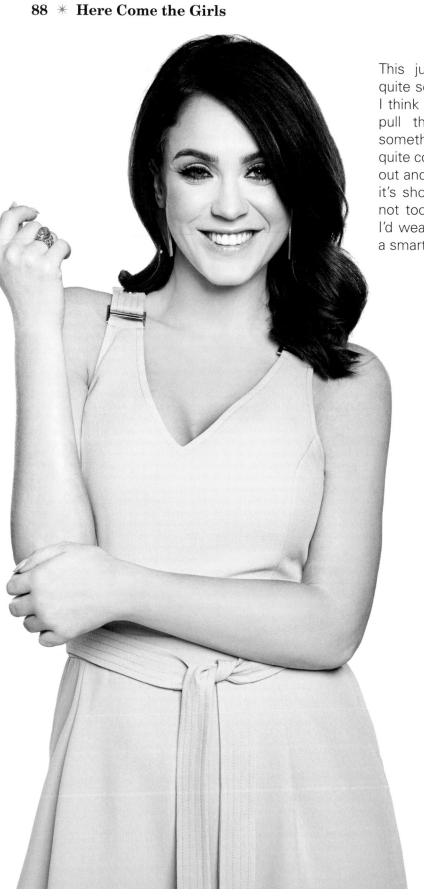

This jumpsuit is demure but still quite sexy. I love the colour pop and I think the shoes and earrings really pull the outfit together. Wearing something bright shows that you're quite confident. You've got your arms out and it's nipped in at the waist so it's showing off your figure, but it's not too over the top and revealing. I'd wear this to a nice restaurant or a smart daytime lunch with friends.

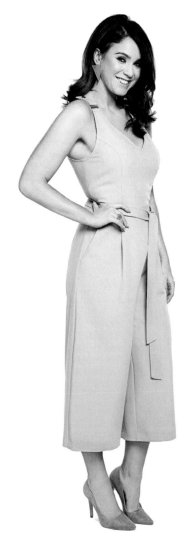

My fail-safe going out make-up looks

How to get contouring right

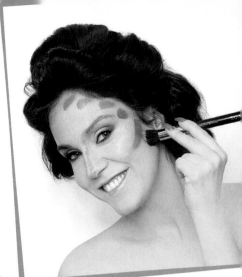

So many people go really over the top with contouring and it can look very unnatural. Bear in mind what looks great in photos doesn't always work in real life!

* If you're a contouring beginner, I would recommend using a powder instead of a cream because it isn't as complicated and it means you can do your usual base routine (see page 27). I have combination-to-oily skin, so I like to use my usual oil-free foundation and then add a powder contour over the top.

    In this picture I'm wearing cream, to show where a make-up artist adds the shading to my face for a full contour look. Attractive, right? But usually I use **Anastasia Beverly Hills' Contour Kit**, which comes in an amazing range of shades. **Barry M's Chisel Cheeks Kit** is a good palette for beginners, as it's got everything you need to start off and isn't too pricey.

* You can't really go too wrong if you contour with a bronzer because it's hard to do a very severe look with it. If I go down this route, I use a matte shade such as **Peaches & Cream Matt Bronzing Powder** as this mimics the skin's natural flat shadows. Save the shimmer for your highlight!

* Apply bronzer or your contour powder just below your cheekbone (suck in your cheeks to find the right spot) using a medium-sized brush and blend, blend, blend using a big fluffy brush. No one wants stripes like a tiger. Apart from a tiger.

* To highlight, I use a light golden shade and apply this around the corner of my eye (tear ducts), along the top of my cheekbones and a tiny bit down the centre of my nose. This makes my skin GLOW! I use **MUA Undress Your Skin in Iridescent Gold**.

* Unless I'm getting my make-up done professionally for a shoot or TV, I don't tend to contour anywhere else on my face apart from my cheeks, and then add my highlights. But you can add shading along your hairline and under your jaw, to really sculpt your face if you want to go for the full Kim K look. The key is to imagine you're sweeping a big letter C onto your face: starting at your temples, swooping round the side of your face under your cheekbones, and then back out again and then around the edge of the jaw. **And then blend. And blend some more.**

✳ To add a bit of colour back into your cheeks, blusher is the way to go. I use **Melba by MAC** to give me a peachy glow, but if you want a high-street alternative check out **Sleek's range of blushers** – they're amazing. I start by smiling to find the apples of my cheeks and then I apply the blush with a round fluffy brush and sweep outwards. This also helps to soften any lines of the contour that stop by the cheek. If you go too heavy, too far up or too far down the cheek, then use a bit of translucent powder over it to blend and soften. If you are unsure whether to go for a shimmer or matte blush, try getting a matte one and then adding your highlighter over it to give it that glow!

How to create a sultry smoky eye

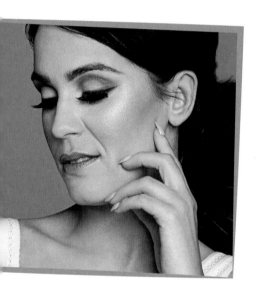

✳ My make-up artists always tell me to start with a base, and **Laura Mercier Eye Basics** is a great one. I use the shade Wheat all over the lid. (**Urban Decay** also have a great range of eye primers, or you could try **Kiko's Eye Base Primer**.) The base is what keeps your eyeshadow on and intensifies the colour.

✳ The next step is to add a medium warm brown into my crease and blend out, then go in with a darker colour and repeat. **Pur Minerals Soul Matte palette** is great because I've got green eyes so burgundy and pinky browns really bring them out. **Sleek's i-Divine palette in Au Naturel** has a similar range of shades. Adding a warm matte bronzer, such as **Bobbi Brown Medium Bronzer**, above my crease stops any harsh lines and blends it softly.

✳ I then add a gel eyeliner (**Kiko's Lasting Gel Eyeliner** is amazing) along the top lash line with a very fine brush. (I get all my brushes from **Crownbrush** as they are a fraction the price of MAC but same quality! Gotta love a bargain.) I then go over the liner with a black shadow to smoke it out. Next I'll run a pencil along the inside of my water line to create even more depth and darkness. I then add a dark pencil liner along my bottom lash line and smoke this out with a plum shadow. You can be a bit messy here as this line doesn't have to be perfect when it's smoky! Same goes for top liner.

✳ If I'm going *out* out, I'll add a touch of golden sparkle to the inner lid (under the socket/crease) and corner of my eyes. You can use your highlighter powder for this.

✳ Finally, I apply a full set of fake lashes and then add individual lashes on top, which is a good layering technique and makes them look full and fluffy. (Always put eyelashes on after you've done the rest of your make-up or you'll end up getting eyeshadow all over them.)

✳ It's best to put lashes on when your eyes are open. If you close your eye, it will scrunch up and when you open it again the lash will be in a different place to where you thought it was going to be!

✳ A great eyelash glue to use is **Duo**. Apply it and then leave it for 60 seconds so it's tacky to the touch before you put the eyelash on. They should be dry and secure pretty much straight away if you do that.

✳ If you're applying individual lashes, it's best to do it with a pair of tweezers. They're a lot more technical so they're much harder to do yourself. You can get lashes that look like they're individual but they're on an invisible strip, and they're much more straightforward. Try **Ardell Wispies**, which I love.

✳ To finish off my eye I'll add a touch of mascara to blend my own eyelashes with the false ones so it looks seamless. My favourite mascara is **Urban Decay Perversion** because the wand is amazing. I also love **Avon's Big Mascara**.

A simple but effective red lip

✳ It's so easy to totally transform a look by changing the colour of your lipstick. I really love red lips for a night out because they look dramatic, and they brighten up an outfit if you've gone for something simple.

✳ If you've got dry lips, try to prepare by exfoliating as much of the dry skin as you can and then adding a lip balm while you do all the other parts of your make-up. Blot your lips before adding lip pencil as the balm can cause products to slide straight off.

✳ I always use a small bit of foundation on my lips as a base. Not only will it keep the lipstick in place, but your lips have their own natural colour so it tones that down.

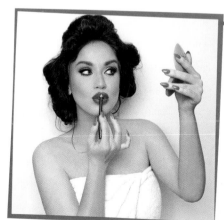
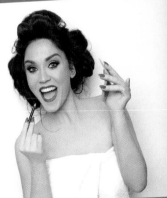

This is totally *how I apply lippie – smiling like a lunatic.*

✳ Next I'll go round my lips with a lip liner and then fill them completely in. This gives a strong colour and makes the lipstick longer lasting.

✳ I love **MAC Lip Pencil in Cherry** and **MAC Ruby Woo lipstick**. You can put Cherry all over the lips and then add Ruby Woo on top for a really dramatic colour that will last no matter how many cocktails you drink. **GOSH Velvet Touch Lip Liner in Simply Red** and **Rimmel Lasting Finish Lipstick by Kate in the shade 111, Kiss of Life** are amazing affordable alternatives.

✳ Another option is to put liner all over your lips with gloss over the top. That way you've got a base colour and you can just keep topping up the gloss whenever you need to. But if you prefer to wear gloss, choose wisely! A lot of lip glosses are too watery and they don't last. **Bobbi Brown**'s are very thick so they really stay on, and the **NYX Mega Shine Lip Gloss** is also fab.

Half up, half down hair (for when you can't make up your mind)

✳ You want to start by curling your hair, using the guide on page 32.

✳ If you want a side parting, section off the front part of your hair and secure in place.

✳ Backcomb the section of the hair that's going up by teasing from the ends to the root. I create the whole shape by backcombing with a brush and using Elnett hairspray to secure it before I put any grips in.

✳ Once you've got the backcombing done it should be solid and stay in place, which means you don't have to use too many clips. Hairpins are easier to hide, but kirby grips are sturdier so they'll keep your hair in place. You should only need about three clips if the shape is secure.

✳ Spray with Elnett and you're away!

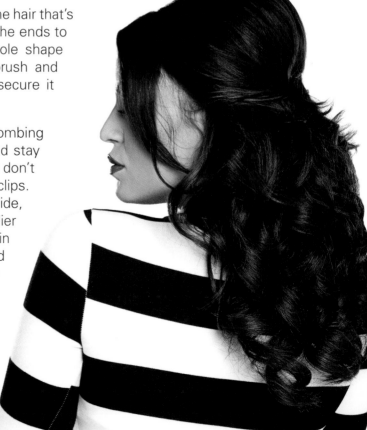

How to have a mint girls' night *in*

My favourite kind of girls' night in is having all the lasses round to mine, putting on comfy pyjamas or a nice pair of trackies, and lazing. We'll watch Netflix or loads of DVDs. (But not scary films because I hate them.)

We always have the two Ps = Prosecco and pizza. We'll get a huge Pepperoni Passion Domino's, loads of hummus, carrot sticks, Doritos, guacamole, salsa, tzatziki, breadsticks . . . basically anything you can dip. If I'm being a bit swanky, I love olives, a good mezze platter with cooked meats and a cheese board. Anything small you can pick at is good because you want to graze all night. Anything you can eat with one hand is good because you need one free for your glass of Prosecco.

I like to spend all night chatting about clothes and lads, doing face packs and generally being really girly. We have never, *ever* had a bad girls' night in. We always have fun and me and the lasses love each other's company.

It's all about the snacks (and the cocktails!)

I've got to be honest, my diet isn't always the first thing on my mind when I have the girls over, but there'll always be someone who wants to stay on the healthy wagon so it's nice to be able to whip something up that'll keep them happy. When it comes to sweet treats though, the diet definitely *has* to go out of the window!

Favourite Girls' Night Movies

- ☞ *She's All That*
- ☞ *Beauty and the Beast*
- ☞ *Erin Brockovich*
- ☞ *Legally Blonde*
- ☞ *Bridesmaids*
- ☞ *Pretty Woman*

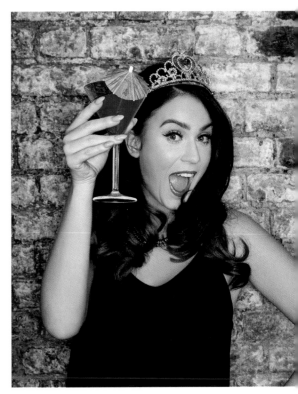

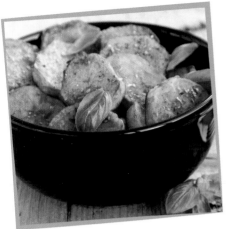

Spicy sumac sweet potato wedges with lemon and lime guacamole (*serves 4–6*)

I love *sweet potatoes!*

I eat loads as they're really good for an everyday healthy lunch. Making them into wedges for a tasty snack is a wicked tip for something simple and healthy that you can just whack in the oven once the girls arrive – you can make the guacamole beforehand, or get the girls to help while you're sorting out the cocktails!

Ingredients

For the wedges

4 medium sweet potatoes (cut into wedges)

2 teaspoons oil (olive or avocado)

1 teaspoon chilli powder

1 teaspoon cumin

1 teaspoon sumac*

For the guacamole

2 ripe avocadoes, (stoned and peeled)

1 red onion (diced)

1 small tomato (diced)

1 teaspoon lemon juice

1 teaspoon lime juice

1 pinch of garlic powder

Method

1. Preheat the oven to 200° C.

2. Place the sweet potato wedges in a bowl and rub in the oil and spices.

3. Spread out the wedges onto a large baking tray and roast for 25–30 minutes.

4. Meanwhile put the guacamole ingredients into a blender to make the dip.

5. Serve the wedges on a plate and the guacamole in a bowl for dipping.

Benefits: *Sweet potatoes are a great source of beta-carotene that can provide antioxidant protection for your skin.*

Avocado is packed full of heart-healthy mono-unsaturated fats that can also keep you feeling full. Homemade guacamole is an easy alternative to shop-bought varieties, which can often contain cream and added sugar.

* Sumac is a tangy spice used in Mediterranean and Middle Eastern cooking. You can find it in most supermarkets.

Strawberry and honeycomb mess (*serves 4*)

Now we're talking! This is so naughty, but delicious and easy to make. Ideal for when you're all crowded on the sofa watching The Notebook *for the 500th time!*

Ingredients

400g strawberries, green leaves removed

200ml whipping cream

1 teaspoon icing sugar

1 teaspoon vanilla extract

2 meringue nests, broken into chunky pieces

1 chocolate-covered honeycomb bar, broken into chunky pieces

Method

1. Save eight strawberries and blend or mash the others to make a smooth strawberry sauce.

2. Put the cream, icing sugar and vanilla in a bowl and whip using an electric whisk until light and fluffy. Gently stir in the meringue, honeycomb and the strawberry sauce to make a swirly pattern.

3. Chop four of the saved strawberries and place in the bottom of four glasses, then spoon in the fruity, creamy mess. Top each glass with a strawberry and chill in the fridge until you're ready to eat.

Girls' night in punch

Ingredients

1 lemon

2 limes

1 punnet strawberries

Pink lemonade

Cranberry juice

Cointreau/Orange Liqueur

Vodka

Method

1. Squeeze the juice of one lemon and one lime into a bowl. Chop the remaining lime into wedges and add to the bowl.

2. Chop up the strawberries and add to the bowl.

3. Pour three cups of pink lemonade and one cup of cranberry juice into the bowl.

4. Add one cup of Cointreau and two cups of vodka.

5. Add ice, mix, ladle out and enjoy!

EASY LIKE SUNDAY MORNING

The morning after the night before.

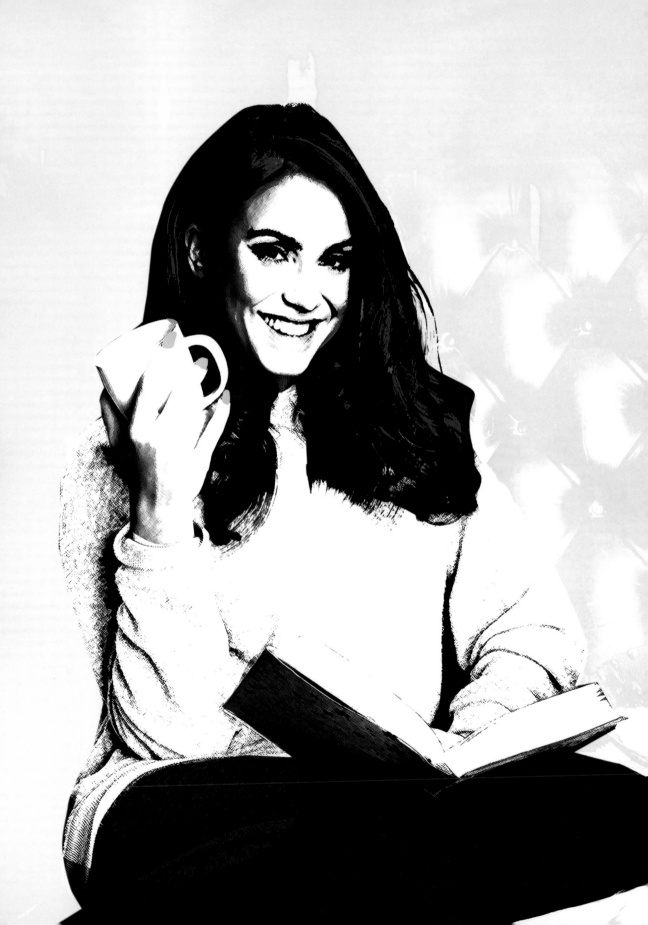

How I like to spend a Sunday when I'm not hideously hungover

How you enjoy a Sunday is all about what you've done on the Saturday night. If I haven't been out, my perfect 'good' Sunday would involve waking up at about 11 o'clock with the sun shining through my window. I go downstairs and have a big but healthy breakfast, like the stuffed mushrooms on page 100. I have a nice glass of orange juice and a green tea and head back upstairs to bed. I sit in bed and watch *Sunday Brunch* on telly. Then I might light some candles, snuggle up under my blanket and read the papers or a book for a while. I just want to completely chill out. Sundays are totally about relaxing and for some people it's the only day of the week they can call a rest day. If I'm feeling really good I'll do a bit of exercise, but nothing too stressful because I want it to fit in with my general laid-back approach to the day.

There are two ways lunch can go on a 'good' Sunday: either I stick to my angelic vibe and have a delicious salad . . . or I go round to my mam's for a roast. The good news is that a roast doesn't have to be bad for you. All the women on Mam's side of the family are curvy, with a tendency to be plump, so she has always been very mindful of how she eats and what she gives to me and Laura. Healthy eating is something that has been impressed upon us since we were young.

If we have a Sunday dinner we'll have chicken, carrots, peas, mashed potato, a couple of Yorkshires and gravy. If you fancy a roast but want to stay healthy, make sure to pile the veggies high and avoid the roast potatoes. (Tricky, I know!)

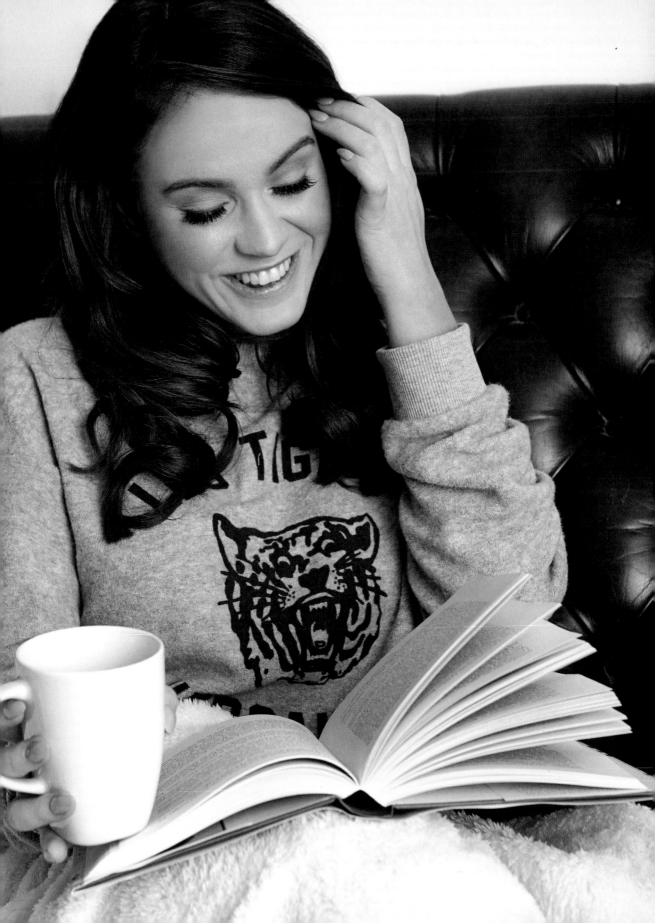

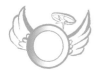

Egg and bacon stuffed mushrooms (*serves 1*)

This is an amazing weekend breakfast that has all the elements of a fry-up, but is actually good for you!

Ingredients

2 portobello or large flat mushrooms

2 thick rashers of bacon (sliced into short ribbons)

2 medium eggs

Sea salt

Black pepper

2 tomatoes (sliced)

Method

1. Preheat the grill to a medium heat.

2. Prepare the mushrooms by gently wiping with kitchen paper and patting dry. Remove the stalks and scoop out the gills with a spoon to create hollows for the eggs.

3. Grill the mushrooms for 5 minutes and allow any moisture to run out.

4. Preheat the oven to 200° C.

5. Place the mushrooms on a baking tray and line each hollow with the bacon ribbons.

6. Crack the eggs carefully into a small bowl. Use a spoon to transfer one yolk to each mushroom. Gradually fill with as much of the remaining egg white as you can fit inside.

7. Sprinkle with a little seasoning and then place in the oven to bake for 15 minutes.

8. Once cooked, serve the mushrooms with the sliced tomatoes.

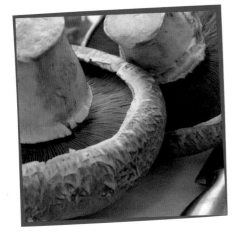

Benefits: *Mushrooms are a low carbohydrate alternative to toast as a breakfast treat, and also a great source of vitamin D for healthy bones. They also provide vitamin B5 for energy and support during stress.*

Eggs are a great source of nutrients – as well as providing protein they give energy-boosting B vitamins and selenium for healthy nails.

Mango and banana detox smoothie

If you have woken up with a bit of a sore head from the night before then necking a fruit smoothie can have you feeling right as rain in no time. This will help rehydrate you and is packed full of vitamin C, which is brilliant at perking you up.

Ingredients

1 mango (chopped into chunks)

1 banana (frozen)

1 teaspoon lemon juice

1 tablespoon chia seeds

½ teaspoon fresh or frozen ginger (chopped)

½ teaspoon turmeric

1 teaspoon coconut oil

1 cup coconut water

1 scoop protein powder (optional)

20 drops of milk thistle tincture (optional)

Method

Blend all the ingredients together until smooth. Simple!

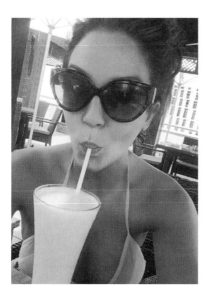

Benefits: *Coconut water is great for rehydration as it is a natural source of electrolytes and tastes great in smoothies. If you're feeling a little delicate then ginger may help to ease feelings of nausea.*

Turmeric can provide antioxidant support for your liver and mango is packed with vitamin C (a water-soluble vitamin that may be lacking if you are dehydrated). Milk thistle can be bought from a health-food shop and is a fantastic herb for liver support if you feel that yours may need a little TLC.

Adding chia seeds and coconut oil helps to provide some good fats and along with the protein powder, will help to stabilise blood-sugar levels.

Rubbed kale salad (*serves 4*)

Kale is one of those fashionable super foods that's everywhere at the moment, and I have to say it's not the most appetising-looking vegetable. But I promise it's worth it if you put loads of delicious flavours with it, like in this salad.

Ingredients

1 packet of kale (approx 200g)

Juice of 1 lemon

1 pinch of sea salt

1 very ripe avocado (peeled and stone removed)

1 handful of pitted olives (sliced)

1 handful of sundried tomatoes (diced)

4 cooked beetroot (diced)

3 spring onions (sliced)

1 yellow pepper (diced)

1 handful of sunflower seeds

1 handful of pumpkin seeds

1 dash of hemp or olive oil

Method

1. Rinse and drain the kale.

2. In a large bowl pour the lemon juice over the kale and sprinkle the sea salt over it.

3. Rub the avocado into the kale, which will soften and wilt.

4. Add the remaining ingredients to the kale, stirring through.

5. Serve on its own, or add some grilled chicken or halloumi for added protein.

Benefits: *Kale is packed full of nutrients, such as vitamin C to boost immunity and vitamin K for healthy bones, as well as the antioxidant beta-carotene.*

Beetroot is a fantastic source of nitric oxide for good circulation and great if you want to get the most out of your gym sessions!

Seeds are packed with essential fatty acids, which are the necessary fats for healthy skin and brain function.

The box sets I love

Saturdays are for seeing your mates and getting drunk, and Sundays are for food, chilling out and family. If you can avoid leaving the house on a Sunday, I definitely would. It's an absolute winner. Sit on the sofa or lie on your bed and watch a box set or a film and completely relax.

Game of Thrones

Because I love the mixture of boobs and dragons. It gets me all fired up.

Scandal

Kerry Washington (and her wardrobe!) is amazing and there's always so much going on.

Modern Family

It makes me laugh so much. I never, ever get bored of watching it.

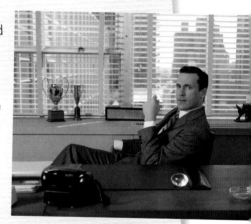

Orange Is the New Black

I loved the first two series. I haven't watched the third series yet but I'm really excited about seeing Ruby Rose in it.

Mad Men

I'm in love with Jon Hamm's character Don Draper – he's a sort.

Criminal Minds

I like anything with a crime theme, and if Derek Morgan isn't Sunday viewing I don't know who is. He's a sort.

CSI

I can sit and watch *CSI* back to back for hours. I never get bored with them.

Suits

It's unbelievable. And full of good-looking men. I am totally hooked.

Luther

It's so, so good. And, of course, it's got Idris Elba in it.

My favourite laid-back Sunday looks

I would love to say I always look like this every time I have a lazy Sunday, but I am *nowhere near* this polished. We couldn't put the pictures of how I really look on a Sunday (even when I'm not hungover) in the book because they'd frighten the life out of you. You'd probably find me wearing a really oversized nightshirt because I like to be free. And no bra. The word 'bra' is a swear-word on a Sunday. You've got to let your boobs live the life and hang out too.

I never wear socks either. They're the sleeping bags of the feet. Your toes feel too trapped and I like my whole body to be able to breathe. Sundays are for slobbing and your feet can't slob in socks. I've got Ugg sheepskin slippers and they're the best investment I've ever made. I'm surprised they don't walk off by themselves because I wear them that much. I love them.

This outfit is perfect for lazing. I do love a onesie, but if I'm feeling really lazy I can't be bothered to take the entire thing off to go to the toilet. You end up sitting on the loo seat naked, which is not acceptable. I love a cosy jumper and joggers for that reason alone.

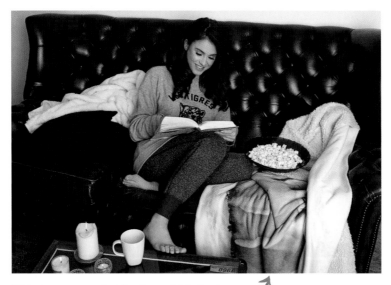

This is my penguin blanket, which I take with me everywhere so I can nap on the go. ↗

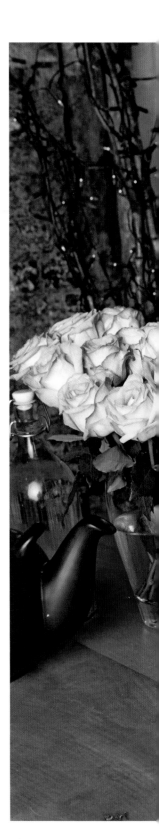

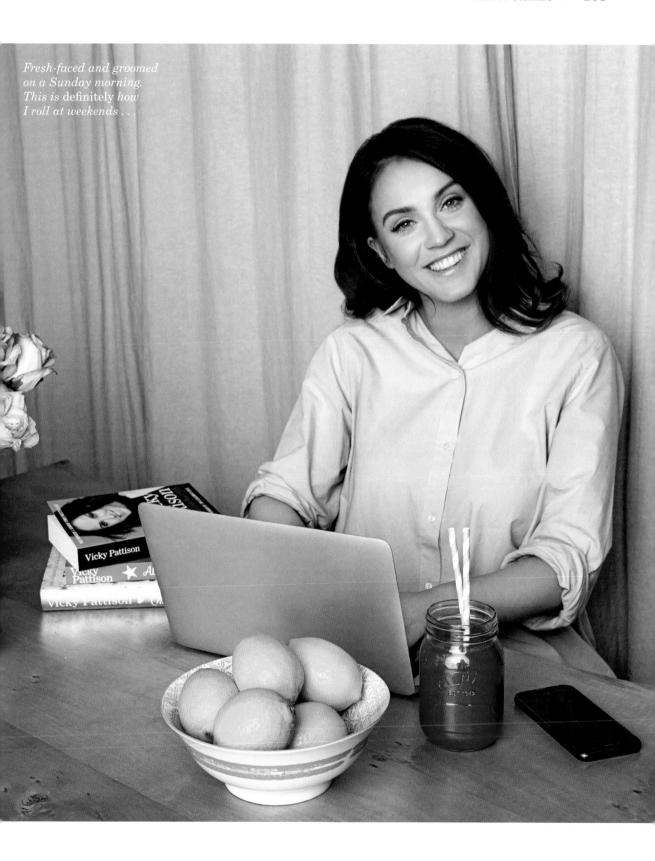

*Fresh-faced and groomed
on a Sunday morning.
This is definitely how
I roll at weekends . . .*

Why Sunday is the perfect day for taking care of your brows

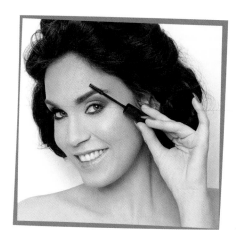

For me, Sundays are a refresh day, so unless I'm going out with my family or friends, I won't wear make-up. You're more likely to find me in a face mask. Well, that's once I take off my make-up from the night before.

If you don't feel confident going completely make-up free I would put on some tinted moisturiser, a bit of mascara and some lip balm. Keep it simple.

As for hair? I don't want it to be in the way when I'm a) eating or b) being sick, if it's been a really big night. I like my hair tied on top of my head in a big bun away from my face. And don't even think about brushing it. The messier the better.

Having said all of that, if you can bear to leave the house, Sundays are the perfect day for getting your eyebrows done because then they've got all day to calm down and no one is going to see you with red eyes. Also, once your brows are sorted the rest of your face instantly looks better, so you can get away with no make-up. I go and get HD brows every two weeks. I get them tinted, threaded, waxed and then plucked. Your eyebrows are measured so they're perfectly symmetrical, and the idea is to get them bigger and more defined.

To make my eyebrows look good for shoots, my make-up artists enhance them by using a gel, like the one by **Anastasia Beverly Hills DipBrow Pomade** or the **Freedom Pro Brow Pomade**. They apply it with a very fine brush and then draw in the individual hairs, so my eyebrows look fluffy – rather than blocky – and then they make them slightly stronger at the ends. Everything gets fixed in place with **GOSH's Clear Defining Brow Gel**, brushing upwards to give effortless fluffy brows. This also clears any face powder that may have got into them. A clear mascara can also do this job really nicely.

Eyebrows on fleek

Eyebrows au naturel

Weekend exercises that you won't mind doing

The weekend is *your* time away from the routine and time restrictions of work, so you have more time to take over your workout. But unless you're training hard for something specific, weekends are also about changing things up and having fun. Rather than just doing your usual gym routine again, why not try going to a class like spinning or body pump, where you can let the instructor lead the session and you can just focus on working hard.

Or if you've had a tough week of training (or a tough week in general!), the weekend might be a good time to go to a yoga or pilates class. You might want to finish this up with a swim and some relaxing time in the sauna or steam room. Taking this time to relax and allow your body to recover will mean you are ready to hit it hard again the following week. Recovery is just as important as training.

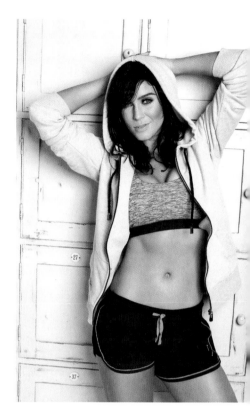

My not-so-good Sunday

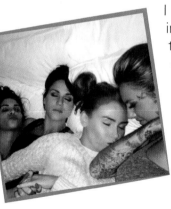

I usually wake up after a big night out with three of the lasses in my bed. We'll be like a human jigsaw. There'll be a kebab on the floor and I'll be gasping for a drink and a fry-up or some other sort of horribly unhealthy breakfast – maybe even a McDonald's. We'll be pretzelled together arguing over who's going to go to the Drive Thru, and knowing we'll be getting pizza later too.

Sometimes I actually prefer a bad Sunday to a good Sunday. I don't know if that's because I've done more bad ones and I'm well practised at them, or whether it's because I can use it as an excuse to be even lazier.

I don't feel guilty about slobbing around all day with a hangover because I know I'm not capable of doing anything else. But if I'm not hungover, sometimes I do feel like I should be at least *trying* to do something instead of lying in front of the TV.

You basically know that if you're going out on a big Saturday night, you're sacrificing Sunday and it's not going to be in any way productive. For me a Saturday night out with the girls is always going to win, so Sunday takes the hit.

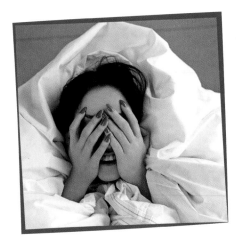

A hungover Sunday with your friends laughing about what you did the night before is all part of the fun. My mates and I will sit and grief each other and howl. We'll spend ages swapping stories about what happened in the toilets or who tashed on with who.

My ultimate bacon sarnie (*serves 2*)

If you're feeling really delicate, you might need to get someone else to make this for you. But it'll be worth it, I promise!

Ingredients

6 bacon rashers

6 cherry tomatoes

2 teaspoons maple syrup

1 small avocado, cut in half and stone removed

2 teaspoons mayonnaise

Squeeze of lemon juice

4 thick slices bread, white, Granary or wholegrain – your choice

Method

1. Preheat the oven to 200° C and place a sheet of foil on a large baking tray. Put the bacon and tomatoes on the baking tray in the oven for 15 minutes. Take the tray out of the oven and put the tomatoes in a bowl – they should be starting to collapse.

2. Brush both sides of each slice of bacon with maple syrup and put the tray back in the oven for another 3 minutes or until the bacon is crisp and sticky.

3. While the bacon is cooking, scoop the avocado out into a bowl and mash with the mayonnaise and lemon juice.

4. Spread the avocado mixture over two slices of bread, then place the bacon on top. Smash the tomatoes and arrange on the bacon then top with the remaining bread to make two sandwiches. Press down gently and cut each sandwich in half.

Bloody Mary vitamin C blast

Sometimes a bit of hair of the dog is the only thing that will sort you out! The vodka in this is optional, if you don't think you can face it!

Ingredients

Salt

Black pepper

1 lime

2 large oranges

1–2 shots of vodka, optional

Worcestershire sauce

Tabasco

1 Stick of Celery

Method

1. Add 1 teaspoon of salt and pepper to a bowl Rim a large glass with a lime wedge.

2. Dip the glass into salt and pepper so the glass rim is evenly spread with both. Fill the glass with ice.

3. Add the juice of 1 orange and your vodka. Add 3 dashes of Worcestershire sauce. Add 3 dashes of tabasco sauce.

4. Add the celery stick, then the orange and lime wedges. Top with black pepper.

5. Sip away your hangover.

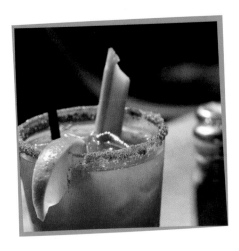

I like everything a hungover Sunday involves, *apart from the actual hangover.*

I'll stay in bed until at least midday (only leaving for supplies) and once I'm 'up', I'll then position myself on the sofa with my blanket and whoever is around, and I'll stay very still and watch anything and everything. Nothing will be done personal-hygiene-wise apart from brushing my teeth, and maybe a bath last thing at night if I can be bothered.

Ten amazing Sunday afternoon films you should watch

You basically want a film to laugh or cry a hangover out of you, keep you entertained, or provide a very handsome man to look at. Anything with Tom Hardy or Denzel Washington is a winner, but never, ever watch *The Green Mile*. Or anything with Tom Hanks in it for that matter, because all of his films are sad, and hangovers are miserable enough.

At about 5 o'clock when I'm starving again, I'll order a Domino's. I'll have a large Pepperoni Passion, chicken strippers, wedges, a large bottle of Diet Coke and cookies for afters. (By the way, exercise is a total no-no with a massive hangover. If you can manage it do some light yoga. Or alternatively do some Domino's yoga, which involves reaching for the Pepperoni Passion and then stretching out for the garlic bread. Breathe into it, exhale and chew. The absolute most amount of physical exertion you do on a hungover Sunday should be walking to the front door to collect your take-away if you can't get someone else to do it for you.) I'll work my way gradually through my feast until about 10 p.m. when I'll fall asleep on the sofa before dragging myself off to bed.

So, in fairness, I haven't wasted my day at all. How can eating pizza and watching TV be a waste?

- *Dirty Dancing*
- *Footloose*
- *Love Actually* (it's not just for Christmas)
- *The Hangover* (fitting)
- *Finding Nemo*
- *Three Men and a Baby*
- *The Notebook*
- *Frozen*
- *Gangster Squad*
- *Zoolander*

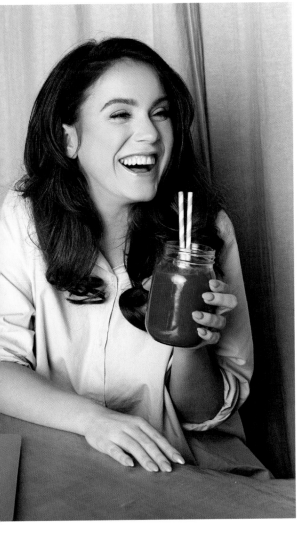

Back to school blues . . .

For me, Sundays are for four things – whether you're hungover or not:

✳ Lie-ins

✳ Family

✳ Sunday dinners

✳ The Sunday night panic at around 8 o'clock

There is nothing more annoying than that feeling you get when your Sunday is coming to an end and you know you've got to get back to reality on the Monday. That pre-work fear hits everyone – it's exactly the same feeling you had when you were a kid and you knew it was school the next day. It's horrible, and it feels really unfair that we never outgrow it! Nowadays, I do my best to minimise the panic by reflecting on the amazing week I've had and the people I've seen and the things I've done. I'll go through my phone and look at pictures of a girls' night out I've had or something lovely I've bought myself, and that cheers me up.

Then I start to plan things for the week ahead and make sure I've got something to look forward to, whether that's meeting up with mates or doing some shopping.

Sunday night should be when you get everything organised for the week ahead. Don't get down about the fact that Monday morning means work. Instead think about that Tuesday-night cinema trip you've got planned with the girls. Always remember that better days are coming, and they're called Saturday and Sunday.

GOAL GETTER

You can do anything you put your mind to!

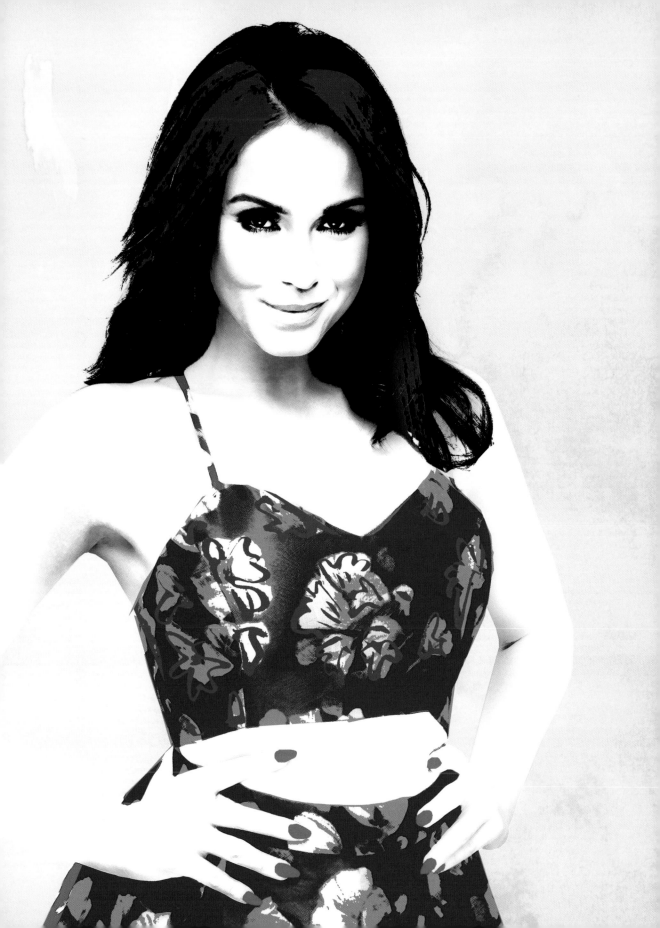

Make a list

I wrote these two goal lists on my phone at the beginning of 2015 and 2016, and I love looking back on them and seeing what I can tick off. These are the genuine lists!

What I want to achieve 2015:

✶ *I'm a Celebrity Get Me Out of Here*

✶ *Judge Geordie* series 2 and 3 (maybe 4)

✶ Number 1 bestselling novel

✶ Contract for 3 new books

✶ Captain of a panellist show

✶ Regular TV presenting on a mainstream channel

✶ *The Xtra Factor*

✶ *FHM* cover

✶ Taking Mini V nutrition into stores and introducing a subscription model

✶ Column

✶ My clothing to be sold on ASOS

✶ *Women's Health* cover

✶ The VIP Collection to launch in Australia

✶ To be a millionaire

✶ Be the face of a big gym brand

✶ Make my own one-off documentary

✶ To be happy

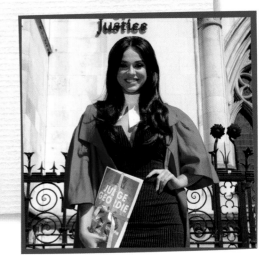

What I want to achieve 2016:

✳ Own 3 properties (including one in London/ down south and possibly a holiday home)

✳ My own chat show (Alan Carr style!)

✳ Regular *Loose Women* panellist and ITV staple

✳ To be happy

✳ Another *Times* number 1 bestseller with my autobiography or lifestyle book

✳ Be a guest on Alan Carr

✳ Team captain on a panel show

✳ Fake tan, hair, perfume, eyelashes . . .

✳ Website to be up and running and a really useful tool for my businesses

✳ New calendar

✳ I want to look into acting

✳ GET INTO DOCUMENTARIES IN A BIG WAY! Professor Green/Reggie Yates style! Big issues that affect young girls that most people are just ignoring, refusing to talk about or discussing with adults or the people it isn't affecting!

✳ A lot of charity work, Spencer's Project, Operation Smile with Duncan, Iceland trek.

✳ An ongoing relationship/campaign with Ann Summers

✳ Present at the MTV EMAs

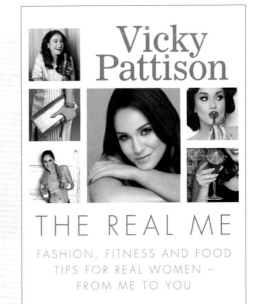

Vicky Pattison

THE REAL ME

FASHION, FITNESS AND FOOD
TIPS FOR REAL WOMEN –
FROM ME TO YOU

Fingers crossed!

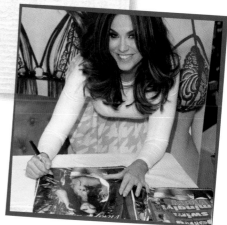

How to get what you want, even when it feels a bit impossible

When I look back at my lists they make me smile because my dreams are so big. And yet I've managed to achieve so many of them, which is incredible.

When I signed with my new agents, Gemma and Nadia from Mokkingbird, in 2015, they asked me to send them a list of what I wanted to achieve. I sent them my goals and I honestly thought they'd send back an email with a load of laughing emojis. Some of the things I wrote down, like winning *I'm a Celebrity*, seemed so ridiculous at that point.

But then they emailed me back and said they'd written a list for me that had a lot of the same things on it, so I knew they were on the same page and that they believed in me too. Sometimes the hardest thing can be actually seeing the potential in yourself, and if someone can help you to see that it's amazing.

If I was going to give just *one* piece of advice to anyone it would be to write down your goals. My mam has been constantly on at me to do it for years, and when I've worked with my life coaches, The Speakmans, they

> **If I was going to give just *one* piece of advice to anyone it would be to write down your goals.**

also told me to do it. A study was done by a woman called Gail Matthews at the Dominican University that showed people who write down their goals accomplish much more than people who don't. And she's clearly very clever, so she knows.

Step one in the whole 'realising your dreams' process is that you have to know what you want. You can't go about achieving anything unless you actually know what it is you want to achieve. And then prioritise. You have to figure out what's at the top of your list, and what you'd happily put a bit further down. Whether it's money, spending time with your family, or getting up every day and enjoying what you do, you need to list them in order of what matters most to you. (And yes, 'being happy' was at the bottom of my 2015 list. I'm still learning, okay?)

I couldn't wake up every day and do the same thing, so my priority has never been to be rich or successful or on the front cover of every magazine going. The most important thing for me was that whatever I did as a career kept me interested. I had to do something that held my attention and made me feel excited; otherwise I wouldn't be able to stick to it for long.

I used that as my starting point to discover what else I wanted. I made my list by working out what I enjoyed doing. I've always loved fashion and because of that I was lucky enough to start working with a clothing company. If I hadn't had a genuine interest in clothes or wanted it to become a big thing, I would have gone along with whatever my business partner wanted and I wouldn't have pushed to be more involved with the designs. I wouldn't have *insisted* on great quality fabrics and made sure that I was involved every step of the way, simply because I wouldn't have cared enough. But I wanted it to be such a big success that it went high up on my list. You have to care about something for it to work. If you're complacent, it's doomed to fail.

There are so many things you can be lacklustre about, but you should be passionate about what you do for a living and bettering yourself. It doesn't matter what your goals are, or how big or small, as long as they're important to you.

One of your goals could be as simple as trying something new every month or going to the gym three times a week. Not every goal has to change the world. On the flip side, you could decide you want to invent something life changing or sail around the world in a dinghy. The most important thing is that it really resonates with you.

Feel the fear . . .

As I've got older and more confident my goals have become wilder, but in no way less achievable. If you want to grow and achieve more you should be constantly reaching for the next step. And don't be afraid to be a bit afraid. Your goals should make you apprehensive if you're going to do things you're proud of. They have to be almost ludicrous, and maybe even on the cusp of being almost unattainable.

If you're not scaring yourself a little bit, you're not growing. If you're deliberately writing down things that you know you can achieve easily, you're doing yourself a disservice. Not that the little things aren't important, because they really are, but you should also have a few things on there even *you* think are crazy. Being scared of them doesn't make you a failure. Not writing them down in the first place does. The bigger our dreams are, the more belief we've got in ourselves and the more space we're giving ourselves to succeed.

Your goal list is your own personal list for you and no one else has to see it, so don't hold back. Once it's written down you can't hide from it and that's what makes it so genuinely useful. If you say to your mates one day 'I want to be a model' or 'I want to be a TV presenter' or 'I want to be a heart surgeon', it's just floating in the air. If you don't action it, you haven't lost anything. **If you write it down you give that goal gravity, and that's what will drive you.**

. . . and do it anyway

Don't be afraid to fail, and don't be discouraged if you don't achieve everything you want to the first time around. Anyone who's ever achieved anything great has failed more times than you can ever imagine.

J. K. Rowling is the most incredible example. Everyone knows she got knocked back from every book publisher going before she got a deal for the Harry Potter books and now look at her. Even I've been to Harry Potter World!

Sylvester Stallone is another good example. Very early on in his career he wasn't getting any work whatsoever and he even did a bit of soft porn to pay his rent. He was so broke he sold his dog, a bull mastiff called Butkus, for $50 just so he could survive. He even ended up homeless for a while. When he wrote the script for *Rocky* he was offered $350,000 for the rights, but he refused to sell it unless he could star in the film. No one wanted to cast him because they thought he was 'funny looking'. But he refused to back down, so eventually they relented and the rest is history. (By the way, he got the dog back and Butkus starred in the first two Rocky films #winner.)

So many people will have come close to giving up on their hopes and dreams, and it was the very last door they knocked on that opened for them. Sometimes your darkest times are the ones right before you succeed, and they're the ones you learn the most from.

Everyone has had setbacks. If you speak to anyone who is successful they will have stumbled along the way. It's not about the fact they fell; it's about the fact they picked themselves back up. If you falter you'll only really fail if you don't try again.

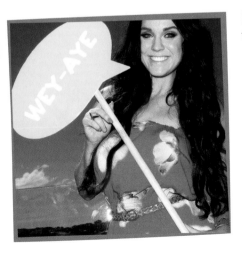

I didn't go seamlessly from working in a call centre to winning *I'm a Celebrity* and getting a job on *Loose Women*. There were a lot of stages in between, and not all of them were easy. There were times when people wouldn't let me into clubs or have meetings with me about TV projects because I was from reality TV. I found myself banging my head against a brick wall at times, but I never once sat and cried and felt sorry for myself. I never wished I'd done things differently or wished I hadn't gone into reality TV. I saw *Geordie Shore* as an amazing platform and I found a way to make it work for me. It was a great way to start out, but I always knew it wasn't where I'd end up.

I wouldn't change my time on Geordie Shore *for anything.*

If you do come across setbacks – which you will, because everyone does – always know that you can overcome them, and take responsibility if you need to. There have been times when I've been my own worst enemy and I've looked around when I've made mistakes and realised that there's no one else to blame. I've had to dig deep and accept responsibility and pull myself back up.

There have been things I've done that have nearly rendered me almost unemployable. Things like my court case (aka 'shoegate') nearly broke me. That was the biggest setback I've ever had. I was three-and-a-half years into *Geordie Shore* and I was finally starting to be press-worthy and get noticed and I went and made the biggest mistake of my life. I risked losing everything.

I was suspended from *Geordie Shore* immediately, and no one had any faith that I'd be asked back. I lost my job, I had a stressful court case and the prospect of a five-year jail sentence.

The court case lasted for six months and every day was hell, so no one can say I didn't have to pay my dues to get success. I had to rebuild my relationship with MTV who didn't trust or respect me any longer, and I had to rebuild my relationship with my family who thought I was a monster. Most importantly, I also had to rebuild my faith and confidence with myself because I'd lost that. I had to work out who I was again because that experience stripped me of everything I thought I knew about myself.

I had to sit down and reflect and work out if being on TV was what I really wanted. Did I want to stay in an industry where I made one mistake and people would sit outside my house and try to take pictures of me and pester my mam? I was followed every time I went to court, and there were people who wanted to see me go to jail because of who I was. It was such a testing time and I had to build myself right back up from the bottom.

As cheesy and clichéd as it sounds, everything I went through made me so much stronger, and it helped me to work out a lot of stuff about myself. I learnt who I truly am and what I'm capable of dealing with. I know I can handle pretty much anything now. I also learnt who my real friends are.

One of my favourite quotes is 'Fake friends are like shadows. They're with you in the sunlight but they'll disappear in the darkness'. And I didn't hear from an awful lot of people for a while after the court case, which made me sad. Those people came back out of the woodwork when I rejoined *Geordie Shore* and my fitness DVD came out, but the damage was done and those friendships have never been the same. I found out what and who really mattered to me over the course of those six months, and who was willing to be there for me whether I was on TV or not.

Sometimes you think a situation will break you and it won't. And you'll learn valuable lessons. I learnt that I wasn't invincible. I was human and I could make mistakes and I would be held accountable for them just like everyone else. I could only pull the duvet over my head for so long before I had to deal with the mistake I'd made, and once I did I knew I was going to be okay.

If you are going through a hard time, speak to someone. Don't go through it on your own. It could be your parents or your best friend or a therapist, but it's about finding whatever helps you.

I know it can be annoying when people say everything happens for a reason, but I guarantee you that six months down the line you'll realise why something happened, so try and see the bigger picture. Nothing is the end of the world and what doesn't kill you makes you stronger.

You're not the first person to face adversity and you won't be the last. Don't beat yourself up too much. If you don't make mistakes you don't grow. You have to have light and shade and go through hard times in order to appreciate the good ones. Don't Chicken Little things. The sky isn't always falling, and sometimes you just have a little bit of rain.

I also believe that sometimes you miss out on something because something even better is coming your way. What's meant for you will come to you, so try not to be too disappointed if you don't get every job you apply for or win every competition you enter. It may just be that something even more amazing is around the corner.

Luck can only take you so far

I totally believe that you can become successful due to luck, but you can't stay there because of it. Kate Moss got discovered at an airport when she was 14 and heading off on holiday with her family. But has she stayed at the top of her game because of luck? God, no! She's worked incredibly hard, been to the right parties, she's schmoozed the right people and always been true to herself. She's kept herself where she wants to be – at the top. She's had heartbreak and she's had setbacks but she's always dusted herself off and got back out there and done better and better each time.

A brilliant opportunity is not enough to forge a career from. It can give you a good start, but you have to have drive and you have to have a plan.

Talent is so important but that can only get you so far. It can give you a step up the ladder, but hard work and dedication are what will get you all the way to the top. It's lovely if you're born with talent but please don't think it's the end of the world if you're not brimming with skills, because it's not everything. If you're talented but bone-idle, I guarantee you that someone who isn't as talented but is really hard working will beat you to a job. It's about hunger and ambition. Don't worry about whether or not you're the best at something because you can become the best. Fake it till you make it.

One thing I would never do, and I would never recommend anyone else to do, is to step on other people to get to the top. There's this idea that to get what you want you have to do something to the detriment of someone else, but it's just not true. It's so much better if you climb the ladder on your own merit using your own skills. And if you're willing to put a hand out and help someone else as you go higher, that's *real* success. Being comfortable enough in your own abilities and achievements that you are able to help others is a real testament to your confidence in your ability to carry on doing well.

The more you do for other people and the more positivity you put out there, the more good karma you'll get back. I'm convinced that's how it works. And you never know when you may need someone to help you out. That shouldn't be your motivation for being good to people because you should want to be a kind person anyway. As my mam taught me, it's nice to be important, but it's more important to be nice.

If someone asks me for a favour I'll always do my best to help them. It's impossible to do absolutely everything, but I will always put myself out and do what I can. Isn't it a lot nicer to look out for each other than to stab each other in the back?

> **One thing I would never do, and I would never recommend anyone else to do, is to step on other people to get to the top.**

We should celebrate each other's successes. There's so much space in this world for everyone to do well and I don't get people who can't be supportive of others. That just makes you bitter.

People have this mentality – especially in the entertainment industry and reality TV in particular – where they think they have to be screaming, slagging people off and causing fights in order to be popular. But it's not about that. It wasn't that way in *Geordie Shore* when we first started the show, but it became like that because it was what was expected of us. But people were actually more interested in the relationships between us, like the bromances between the lads, or when Charlotte cried and I'd hug her. It was the nice stuff people liked.

If you're fixated on or jealous of someone else's achievements you're never going to be happy because you can't measure yourself against someone

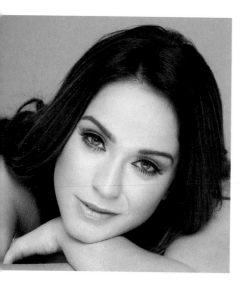

else's success. The only person you should compete with is yourself. Helping someone else achieve their goals isn't going to stop you achieving yours. If anything, the universe will reward you quicker. What goes around comes around and if you're rooting for other people to fail that negativity will rub off on you.

We're all given the same amount of opportunities and it's about what you make of them and how grateful you are and how you treat others. I'm all about women supporting other women too. When I do Woman Crush Wednesday on Instagram, I either do it to get friends more followers or to celebrate other amazing women and appreciate their beauty – inside and out. I do it to build people up. I know it may seem trivial but it makes me feel happy whenever I do it. I believe that little things go a long way.

So to summarise, if you want to achieve your goals . . .

- ✳ **Write them down and prioritise**

- ✳ **Stay positive**

- ✳ **Don't worry about setbacks. They will come and they can be overcome**

- ✳ **Be strong**

- ✳ **Be resilient**

- ✳ **Be determined**

- ✳ **Don't step on other people**

- ✳ **Help people when you can**

- ✳ **Be kind to yourself**

All That Glitters . . . is really hard work, but so much fun!

I've always loved reading and writing, so one of my goals from a really young age was to write fiction. My debut novel All That Glitters *was one of the first things I was able to do off the back of* Geordie Shore *that was truly a passion project.*

When I first started talking to publishers, I wanted to do a novel straight away. My editors at Little, Brown weren't opposed to me writing fiction at some point in the future but they wanted to release my autobiography first, which was a very logical way to go. They wanted to see if I had a fanbase for books.

When my autobiography did really well and I was offered a contract to write two novels, I couldn't keep the smile off my face. It was the proudest moment of my professional career at that point, because no one was expecting it. We got straight to work as soon as the ink was dry. The plan was for *All That Glitters* to be a summer beach read, and then of course my second book, *A Christmas Kiss*, was going to come out in time for the festive season. Both were on really tight schedules and there is no room for deviation in publishing – if you've got a deadline, you have to hit it.

I wanted the books to be of a high standard, funny, heartwarming and easy to read, and I was so lucky to have such a strong team to help me achieve that because I couldn't have done it on my own. (That's another lesson: don't be too proud to accept help and support from others!) I've never hidden the fact that I have help with my books, but I'll have words with anyone who tries to suggest I've not been involved in the writing. I work bloody hard on all my books, and I poured my heart and soul into both novels. My absolute favourite part of the process is brainstorming the story and coming up with all the characters. I get really into deciding how they look, what their personality's like and I *love* choosing their names! I get locked into a room at Little, Brown with my team and a pile of snacks, and we don't come out until we've nailed an amazing storyline!

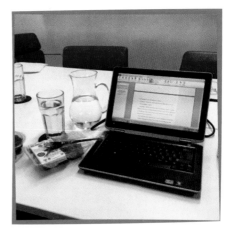

The glamorous life of an author!

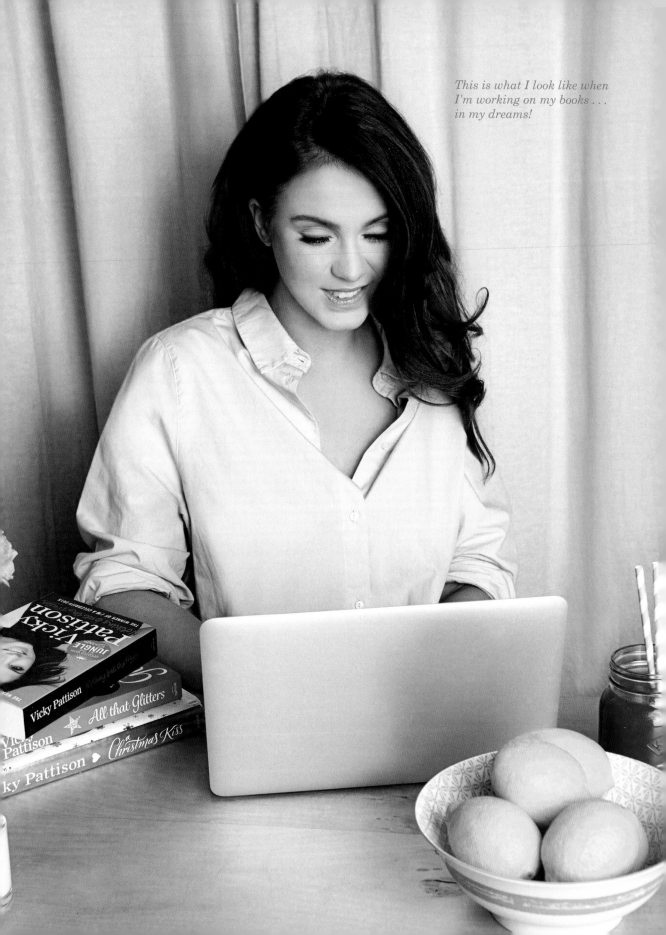

This is what I look like when I'm working on my books . . . in my dreams!

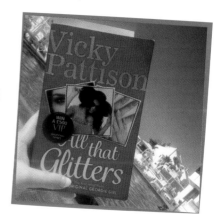

I had such a sense of achievement when I finally held a finished copy of *All That Glitters* in my hand. Seeing anything you've worked on come to life is amazing, and I was like an excited child. I knew how much work had gone into it, so it meant everything to me. Getting the novels in bookshops involved a lot of hard work from everyone, but I knew it was worth it when people started sending me pictures of them reading *All That Glitters* around the pool on holiday.

Writing novels is something I hope to continue doing because even though it can be tough at times, I absolutely love it. And as I've said before, if you don't push yourself, you don't grow. I really hope to spread my wings in the literary world and I don't just want the fact my name is on the book to be the thing that sells it. I want all of my books to be brilliant reads that just happen to be written by me; I want people who've never seen me on telly to pick up one of my books and enjoy it, without knowing a thing about who I am. I understand that I'm very wet behind the ears and I've got a long way to go, but I'm so grateful for the opportunity.

Fancy a cheeky read of my literary masterpiece? Read on for the first chapter of *All That Glitters* . . .

Prologue

Issy Jones felt fat warm tears sliding down her cheeks. She grasped her dad's hand tightly; it felt cold and unfamiliar. She barely recognised the man lying in front of her on the hospital bed, multiple tubes and wires attached to him. He had the same familiar dark hair and even features she knew so well, but his face was pale and so, so still. She squeezed his hand tighter as the machines continued to bleep around them.

'I promise I will do anything, absolutely anything if you get better, Dad,' Issy whispered, unsure if he could hear her.

'And I'll never leave you again. Just be all right. Please, Dad.

Please.'

Still holding her dad's hand, she slumped down in the hard, uncomfortable hospital chair next to him and rested her head on his arm, remembering how safe she used to feel when he hugged her as a child. She didn't want to let go, afraid if she did she would lose him forever, and she wouldn't be able to bear that. Even the thought of it brought tears to her eyes and Issy breathed deeply, trying not to despair.

It had all happened so suddenly. Only the day before she'd been working on an assignment at her hairdressing college in London, when she got a call from her brother, Zach, shakily telling her that their dad had suffered a heart attack. She'd dropped everything, rushed to the station and caught the first train she could home. A tear-filled three hours later, Zach had met her at Manchester station and had warned her that their dad was in a bad way.

But nothing could have prepared her for seeing him look so frail.

The man in the hospital bed, wired up to machines, wasn't the gentle giant who had cared for her growing up. Issy's dad was a tall, handsome, muscular man, the years working in his garage had seen to that, but the figure in front of her seemed smaller and older than the man she knew.

The change in him had been so shocking her legs had almost given way when she'd first seen him. Zach had grabbed her to stop her from falling, and then held her while she cried. Her mum, Debs, who always had something to say, was silent as they stood together watching his chest rise and fall.

The three of them stayed by his bedside all night. At some point Zach had dropped off to sleep, and while he softly snored Issy and her mum had talked for hours, trying to keep each other's spirits up. But it hadn't worked. The fear was visible on their faces and in their trembling voices. Neither of them had wanted to think about what life would be like without the man who made them feel safe.

Issy took another deep breath, reminding herself to stay positive.

'Issy?' a husky voice said. She lifted her head off her dad's arm and tried to blink the tears away.

'Dad?' She wondered if she had imagined it. She felt a rush of hope as she saw his eyes flicker towards her.

'Isabelle, are you crying?' His voice was croaky and full of concern.

'Of course not,' Issy replied, brushing her cheeks. 'What's with the Isabelle? You only call me Isabelle when I've done something wrong.'

'I don't want you crying, kiddo. Help me out and find someone who can tell me what's really going on here, will you . . . ?'

'I'll call someone and get some help,' she said, getting up and reluctantly letting go of his hand.

She walked out into the corridor and took several long, deep breaths. A few hours after he'd been admitted the doctors had declared her dad 'stable', but she hadn't believed them. Not until now. This was what she'd been praying for, yet she still couldn't quite believe it.

After steadying herself, Issy grabbed the first nurse she saw, a young woman about her own age who looked perky enough to be early in her shift, so when Issy explained that her dad was awake she followed right after. She was the only member of the family left at the hospital and felt like a child, hopelessly out of her depth. Her brother had gone to check on the garage their dad owned and ran, while her mum had gone home for some rest. She wished they were both here.

When Issy followed the nurse back into the room, her dad had barely moved but his eyes were wide open and there was a sense of awareness about him. Relief flooded through her. He really was going to be all right.

'You gave us quite a fright, Mr Jones,' the nurse said sternly but with a smile.

'Yes you bloody well did,' Issy added, flashing him a beaming smile.

'Hey, love, sorry about the fright, but please, call me Kev.' He winked at the nurse.

'Really, Dad? One minute you're at death's door the next you're putting a shift in with a nurse!' Issy shook her head but she was still grinning.

Before he could reply the door to the ward burst open and her mum ran into the room clutching her yapping little dog, Princess Tiger-Lily, followed closely by Zach. She immediately launched herself on her husband, showering him with kisses.

'Debs!' Kev spluttered.

'You can't have dogs in here,' said the nurse sounding shocked and angry. 'We don't allow animals in the hospital and your husband is still very ill.'

'You shouldn't have brought her in here, love,' Kev said quietly. It was an effort to lift his hand but he gently stroked the side of Debs's face.

'I did try to stop her,' Zach said, turning his attention to the flustered nurse. He mouthed a silent 'sorry' at her and she visibly melted. Issy rolled her eyes. Her brother could charm his way into a nun's pants.

'Oh for God's sake, he's alive, that's all that matters. And surely you know how important pets are for patient rehabilitation?' Debs said, wagging a finger at the nurse.

'Just be careful. There are a lot of wires,' she simpered, eyes still fixed upon Zach. 'I'll go and see where the doctor's got to.'

'You do that, love,' Debs replied with a smile before carefully placing Princess at the foot of the bed and launching herself onto Kev again.

'Mum, you'll give him another heart attack carrying on like that,' Zach half-joked.

The nurse backed out of the room, her gaze firmly fixed on Zach, who had been pretending not to notice.

Issy stood in the small, grey hospital room surveying her family. She couldn't believe all their happiness had nearly been taken away from them. A rush of pure love filled her as she looked around at them all; her dad, her mum, Zach, even Princess Tiger-Lily, right now she'd even forgive all those times her barking interrupted a much-needed Saturday morning hangover lie-in.

It wasn't normal, it was quite far from normal, but they were hers and she loved everything about them. She meant what she had said before her dad had woken up; she would never leave them again.

Chapter One

THREE YEARS LATER

'So, what are we doing today, Vi?' Issy asked, wielding a pair of scissors and standing behind Violet, one of her regulars. They were in A Cut Above, her mum's hairdressing salon in Salford, on the outskirts of Manchester. It was the most popular salon in the area but that was because most of the clients belonged to the blue rinse brigade. Although there were a few younger customers, it wasn't exactly what you'd call edgy, and Issy longed to get her creative hands on people who wanted more than a trim and tint. Issy had asked what Vi wanted, already knowing the answer. She'd known Vi and many of her mum's other clients since she was a little girl.

'I just want a little bit off, duck. Not too short, mind. I don't want to look like a poodle,' Vi replied. Issy nodded. With her tightly permed white hair, no matter what she did Vi always ended up looking like a poodle.

'Of course not, Vi, God forbid,' Issy said, smiling warmly at Violet in the mirror.

Issy got to work on Vi's hair when suddenly a wave of nostalgia hit and she was catapulted back to her days at The Hair Academy. It felt like a lifetime ago that she'd walked away from her course.

The Hair Academy was the most illustrious hairdressing college in the UK, and Issy had worked her arse off to get a place on one of their courses. They only took a handful of students each year so competition was fierce, but back then Issy was full of confidence – and had the talent to back it up. Prior to her dad's heart attack, she'd been so driven and ambitious. Whether she ended up styling hair for magazine shoots or working backstage at fashion shows – one way or another she had been determined to make a name for herself.

It was a far cry from where she was now.

Issy looked around the salon. She'd practically grown up here – hairdressing was in her blood. Her mum had started teaching her how to style hair when she was barely a teenager. She'd practised on dummy heads, swept up hair, made notes – whatever it took to learn the trade. As a young girl, it had amazed Issy that people could come into the salon looking pretty ordinary and leave feeling amazing. Hair was powerful, she truly believed that. Hairdressing was about more than just the physical, there was a psychology to it too. People poured their hearts out when they sat in the hairdresser's chair and Issy understood that she was much more than a pair of scissors to them, they put their trust into her when they sat down in her chair.

Issy shook her head to dispel her nostalgia and tuned back into Vi's chatter about her latest ailments. Issy missed the glamour and the creative challenges of The Hair Academy, but her mum's salon had heart and the clients were important to her. They needed her and so did her family. Readjusting to living at home again had been hard but Issy had never once doubted that leaving her course and coming back to Salford had been the right decision.

A melodic hum of chatter filled the air. A Cut Above was a medium-sized salon and as well as Issy and her mother, Karen and Brenda, two other stylists, also worked there. Alice, their trainee, completed their small team and though at the moment she was shampooing, sweeping up hair and making tea, she was bright and good with the clients so Issy knew it wouldn't be long before she had the skills and confidence to start tackling cuts on her own. It was how they'd all got their start.

'Thanks, Alice,' Issy said as Alice delivered a cup of milky tea to Violet. Alice smiled back at Issy and said hello to Vi, before going off with her broom.

There was a commotion as the door opened and Issy turned to see Zach walking through the salon. He'd clearly come from the garage – it was just around the corner so they were always popping in and out – as he was wearing his oil-covered overalls, and his cuffs were rolled up to reveal his full-sleeve tattoo. Since their dad's heart attack, Zach had taken charge of all the manual labour at the garage and Issy's dad had taken a step back and focused on the office work. Kev insisted that he didn't mind the change but Issy secretly thought that he did miss getting his hands dirty.

'Ooo,' Vi said, turning her head suddenly and almost losing an ear in the process. Issy pulled her scissors quickly out of harm's way, she knew how Vi could get around Zach, or any young man, in fact. 'Zach, hi!' Vi waved flirtatiously as Zach made his way over to them.

'Hey, gorgeous,' he said to Vi. She blushed like a girl a quarter of her age and Issy shook her head.

At six foot two, Zach shared the same dark hair as Issy and their dad. He was definitely a good-looking lad, and had been for as long as Issy could remember. She'd been one of the most popular girls in school simply because girls thought they could get close to Zach through Issy. And he was still one of the fittest lads in Salford – not that Issy would ever tell him that. Zach definitely didn't have confidence issues.

'What are you doing here?' Issy asked.

'I had a few minutes so I thought I'd pop in for a sunbed.'

'Are you going to be naked?' Vi asked hopefully.

Issy's eyes sparkled with amusement. 'Vi, you're old enough to be his nan,' she rebuked.

'I am not,' Vi replied indignantly.

'No, Vi, I wear boxers in there,' Zach said conspiratorially, lifting his T-shirt to snap at the waistband of his Calvin Kleins and exposing a strip of muscular stomach as he did so. 'Got to protect little Zach!'

Issy looked around the salon. Alice was almost the same colour as Issy's crimson nails, Vi was grinning from ear-to-ear and Karen couldn't keep her eyes off Zach's groin.

'Right, that's enough,' Debs shouted, coming out from the back fresh from cleaning the sunbeds. 'Zachary Jones, get into that sunbed and leave everyone else to cut hair.' Zach threw Vi a final cheeky wink and then disappeared.

Vi chatted non-stop about Zach for the rest of her hair-cut. Issy shared a smile with her mum who was sorting out accounts and manning reception. Zach had taken on the lion's share of the work at the garage for the last three years and she was proud of him – despite the fact that he flirted with old ladies. Although in fairness he flirted with everyone and everything – dogs, pot plants, a packet of chocolate digestives. Nothing and no one was immune to Zachary Jones's charms.

Issy was just finishing up with Vi when the salon door banged open again and her father appeared.

'Hello, gorgeous,' Debs said, coming round from the reception desk to kiss her husband, wrapping her arms around him in a display of affection that made Issy feel like an awkward teenager.

'Hi, love.' Kev looked around the salon and smiled. 'Hi, ladies.'

'Two handsome men in one day,' Vi said. 'I shall never recover.' Issy thought, not for the first time, that despite her age, Vi was still a saucy old flirt.

'What other handsome man?' Kev asked, sounding perplexed.

'Your son, love. He's having a sunbed.'

'That's where the bugger got to. He said he had to pop out for teabags half an hour ago. I should have known where he'd be.' Kev looked annoyed but deep down he was more amused by Zach than angry. Father and son were like peas in a pod, but Zach was the new generation, for sure. He took care of himself in a way that Kev could never understand. Zach was a man's man, but a well-groomed one.

At that moment Zach reappeared, a few shades darker than when he'd come in.

'Bollocks!' he said on seeing his dad. He ducked down behind Vi's chair. 'Protect me, Vi.'

'Any time, love,' Vi said, a wicked glint in her eye.

Zach laughed. 'What are you doing here, Dad?' he asked, standing up but still keeping a good distance.

'Well, I was hoping for a word in private with our Issy,' he said, shuffling awkwardly from foot to foot.

'What about?' Debs asked.

'Yes, what about?' Vi repeated. Vi loved coming to the salon – it was better than an episode of *Coronation Street*.

Issy jumped in. Just because it was a family business didn't mean that everyone got to hear all their business. 'Give me five minutes and I'll come and see you – Vi's my last cut of the day.'

'Meet me at the café, I could murder a cuppa.' He shot his son a look. 'And Zach, get back to work.'

'Come on, Dad. At least I'm a lovely colour now,' Zach laughed.

'A lovely colour? You're starting to resemble a bloody tea bag, you big girl – now get back to the garage, will you?' Kev said, exasperated.

'Oh you really are a lovely colour,' Vi agreed. 'If only you'd show me your tan lines.'

'Bloody hell, Vi!' Debs shouted, but with a laugh. 'Boys – out, any more of this and Alice'll be sweeping up fainting pensioners instead of hair.'

Issy pulled her black cardigan around her as she walked towards the café. It was cold, but she didn't have far to go. She pushed open the door and saw her dad, sitting at a corner table, reading a newspaper, with two mugs of tea in front of him. She smiled at the woman behind the counter and made her way over.

'Hiya,' she said, sitting down and pointing at his mug.

'There better not be any sugar in that tea?'

'Course not,' Kev replied, looking guilty. Since his heart attack, Issy had been on a one-woman mission to make sure her dad stayed healthy. She resisted the urge to take a sip to check. He was pretty patient about her bossing him around but she didn't want to push her luck.

'So, what's going on?' Issy had a sudden thought. 'Is everything OK? Is it your heart?' However many years passed, Issy didn't think she'd ever stop worrying about her dad having another heart attack.

'No, it's nothing like that. I'm fit as a fiddle, promise.' Issy relaxed back into her chair. 'Am I in trouble then?'

She smiled at her dad the way she always did when she needed to get round him.

'No, you're not in trouble. I just . . . well . . . OK . . . Look, there's something I wanted to talk to you about.' Kev looked awkward as he shuffled in his seat. 'The thing is, well, you've been back at home for three years now.'

Issy frowned. What was this all about?

Kev took a deep breath before continuing. 'Here's the thing. Three years ago you were in London, following your dream, full of ideas and ambition. We both know why you came home but I'm not sure I know why you're still here.'

'Dad, what are you getting at?' Sometimes her dad took for ever getting to the point. Cars, rather than conversation, were Kev's strong point.

'I just want to make sure that you're happy, you know, living at home and working at the salon. Is cutting old ladies' hair really what you want?'

'There are worse jobs,' Issy said defensively.

'I know that, and your mum's salon is grand. But you've always wanted more. You've got your mum's talent but we always wanted more for you as well. Once me and your mum met it was all marriage, babies and bloody dogs. Wish I'd put me foot down and insisted we got a cat.'

'Dad. I have no idea what you're talking about. Is this about me or Princess?' Issy looked her father straight in the eye.

'Bloody hell, Issy. Can't I have a proper conversation with my daughter?'

'Sure.' Issy smiled sweetly. 'And if I knew what this was about then I could join in with that proper conversation.'

Kev looked cross at first and then started laughing. He should've known better – Issy always cut to the chase.

'Here's the thing. It's time for you to put yourself first,' Kev said gruffly. 'You kept this family together when I was ill. Now it's time I did something for you, and I have a plan.'

'A plan?'

'I saw an advert for a new reality TV show. It's a hairdressing competition and the production company is looking for contestants. The best thing is that it will be filmed in Manchester.'

'A TV show? Are you mad?' Issy loved watching reality TV, she was a hopeless addict, but that didn't mean she wanted to be on it. Of course the 'what if' had crossed her mind, but she couldn't see it. She'd never wanted to be famous.

'You're perfect for it,' Kev said. 'You have the talent for it and you'd still be nearby so you wouldn't even be leaving us really.'

'This show – what is it exactly?' Issy fiddled with a salt shaker as she tried to make sense of what her dad was saying. The idea of it had filled her with an uncharacteristic dread.

'All I know is that it's a competition for hairdressers, it's going to be on TV, and there's some big prize.'

'Well, that's not a lot to go on. It sounds all right but, Dad, a TV show? Come on. They probably wouldn't want me anyway.'

'The thing is . . . that . . . I sort of filled out the application form for you and it turns out they do want to speak to you.' Kev stared at the table as intently as if they were showing an episode of *Match of the Day* on there.

'You did what?!' Issy shrieked. 'Dad, have you gone mad?'

Issy couldn't believe what she was hearing.

'Someone had to do something!' Kev looked annoyed until he saw the panicked look on Issy's face. He picked up his mug and then put it back down again. 'I only did it because I love you,' he said talking to the table again, a blush slowly creeping up his neck.

Issy was silent for a moment. How am I meant to respond to that? she thought.

'I love you too, Dad,' Issy said finally. 'But what's that got to do with some daft TV show?'

'The London thing . . . it was a big deal and you gave it up. For us, for me. I know you felt that you had to prop all of us up and we let you, but only because we thought you'd go back once everything was back to normal.' He smiled, back on more comfortable territory. 'It's time for you to get back to your life and stop living ours.'

'I'm not sure I have it in me any more, it's been too long.' Issy felt confused. Of all the things she could have imagined her dad was going to say, this didn't come close. She didn't know how to react and it was bringing all her unacknowledged fears to the surface.

'Don't be so bloody dramatic, of course you have. You're only twenty-five. You've got your whole life ahead of you.'

'But Dad—'

'This show could open doors for you. Look, you're wasting your talents here and it's not on.' He looked stern and Issy wondered if she was still expected to do as she was told at her age.

'I'm scared, Dad,' she admitted, looking at the table herself now.

'There was a time when nothing scared you.' Kev reached for Issy's hand. 'Where's my brave daughter gone? The daughter who had bigger balls than most of the lads in my garage? Is she still in there?'

Issy laughed, despite herself. 'I don't know, Dad. I need to think about this properly. I'm a little bit blindsided.'

'OK, love, but don't take too long. They won't wait forever.' Her dad looked her square in the eye for the first time since she'd come in. 'The only thing that matters to me is that you're happy. And I don't think you've been truly happy since you moved back home.'

Issy stood up and walked round the table so she could sit next to her dad. She enveloped him in a hug. Kev gave her a squeeze back.

The two mugs of tea were left undrunk.

My favourite non-twatty inspirational quotes

I'm sorry to anyone who follows me on Instagram because I do post quite a lot of inspirational quotes, but they're for my benefit as much as everyone else's.

I love affirmations and if I'm having a bad day, saying something positive to myself repeatedly can really lift my mood and help me to feel focused.

Some of my favourites are:

LET YOUR
HATERS
BE YOUR
MOTIVATORS

Hard work beats talent when talent doesn't work hard

Make today so *amazing* yesterday gets jealous

Trust yourself. You know more than you think you do

IF YOUR DREAMS DON'T SCARE YOU, THEY'RE NOT BIG ENOUGH

Girls tear down other girls whereas women empower each other

My career highlights. Funnily enough one of them involves a jungle

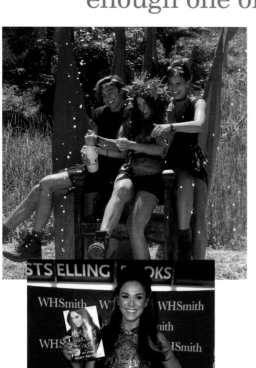

✳ **Going on *I'm a Celebrity* and winning**

Without a doubt one of the best moments of my life. So much changed for me in such a short amount of time.

✳ **Having a *Sunday Times* Number 1 best-seller with my autobiography**

I could not have been prouder of this. I still wasn't that well known at the time but the book sold amazingly well.

✳ **Having the number 1 selling DVD in the entire country with *7 Day Slim***

Another massive achievement. I'd just been through a really tough time and this was my silver lining.

✳ **Being a part of three hit MTV reality shows: *Geordie Shore, Ex on the Beach* and *Judge Geordie***

I had a lot of fun on all of those shows, and getting my own series with Judge Geordie was amazing.

✳ **Having the courage to leave *Geordie Shore,***

Although leaving was a really difficult thing to do I knew it was the right time for me. Once I'd taken that leap I felt both excited and terrified.

✳ **Landing my first national campaign with Ann Summers**

It's a brand that's about feminine empowerment and being in touch with your sexuality and who you are, which is what I'm all about.

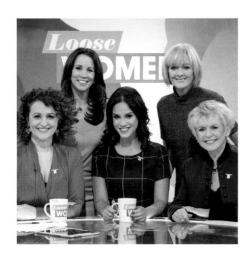

✳ **Getting a regular slot on *Loose Women***

I've always been a huge fan of the show and it was genuinely a dream come true when I become a regular panellist.

✳ **Making my first million**

We're brought up not to talk about money, and maybe me saying this sounds really arrogant . . . but honestly, that was the most unbelievable moment for me. An amazing milestone, and the product of a huge amount of hard work. It means security, which is so important to me.

LIFE'S A BEACH

Get yourself in shape for the holiday of your dreams.

8

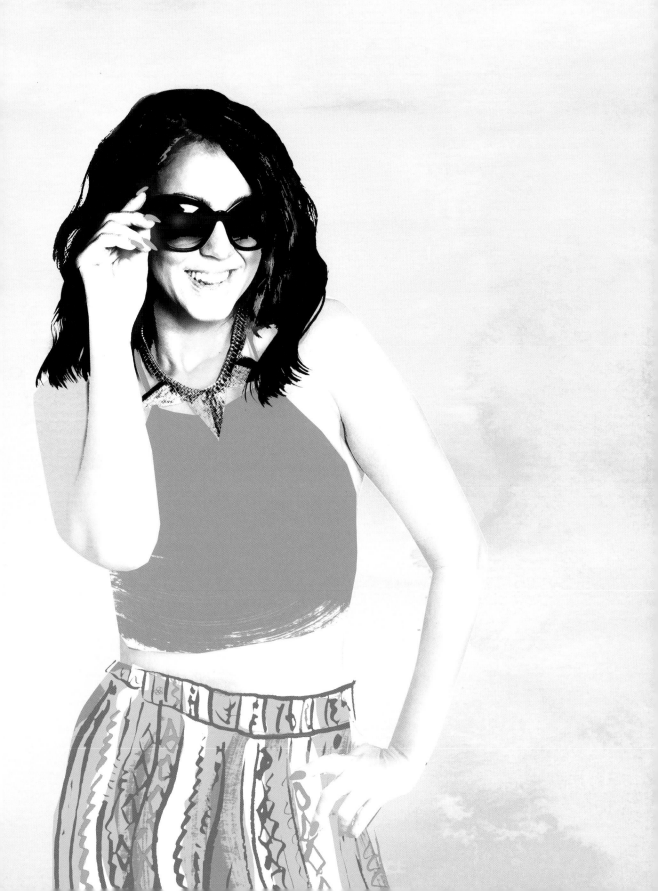

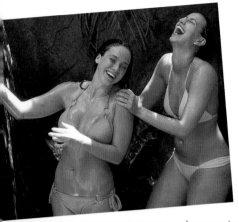

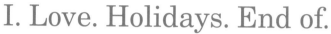

I. Love. Holidays. End of.

I've been lucky enough to go on some amazing holidays over the years, and now I get to travel a lot because of my job, too. I love seeing the world and experiencing different places. I'm a very lucky girl.

The best holiday I've ever had was when I went to Ibiza with the lasses in 2009. We were in some dive hotel that was falling apart, but we had the best laugh. Ibiza will always be my favourite place to visit. I went back with Stephen Bear when we were dating and I saw a totally different side to the party island everyone thinks of. We went to lovely restaurants and watched the sun set – it was so romantic. Another amazing trip was when I went to the Riviera Maya in Mexico with my family. It was beautiful weather, it had gorgeous restaurants and it was so chilled. Mexican people are so friendly and welcoming.

Sydney in Australia is absolutely beautiful, too. It's got that real city vibe in the centre. People rushing around in suits and there are gorgeous designer shops and amazing bars. Then if you drive for twenty minutes you're at Bondi Beach and everyone's chilling and walking their dogs and surfing.

I haven't had many terrible holidays but I did once go to Paris with a boy I didn't like simply because I wanted to go and see the city. I knew I wasn't that keen on the lad and it was a mistake going to a place I'd wanted to see so badly with someone I barely knew. Paris isn't ruined for me because of that experience and I've been back loads of times since and I absolutely love it, but I'll never shake the feeling that I wish I'd gone there with someone special the first time. Special places should be enjoyed with special people.

When I did my season in Magaluf, I initially went out there on holiday with the lasses to see if I could find work, and it was both hilarious and awful. By the end of my trip I'd found a job in a bar, so I was going to stay and move into an apartment with a girl who also worked there. When I went to put my case in the apartment my new flatmate wasn't home to let me in, and because I'd dragged it up a massive hill I couldn't be bothered to take it all the way down again. I was also running late for work, so I shoved it in a store cupboard . . . where it promptly got stolen.

Everything I'd taken to Magaluf was gone. I was so devastated. My mates were furious, so they marched me to the apartments and knocked on every single door until they found it. It turned up in the top floor apartment and the two geezers who lived there pretended to be really confused about how it got there . . . All of my expensive stuff had been taken, like my designer watch and sunglasses. They'd probably sold them or something. But I refused to let them ruin my season and I was determined to stay and have a good time anyway.

Everyone who worked in the bar where I'd found a job did a whip-round for me and I was so touched when they handed me over an envelope with money in it. That showed what great people I was working with and I had the best time of my life over there.

Having a bikini panic? Get your trainers on and get busy

Try my pre-holiday gym programme, which is a timed and structured plan to get your body ready for the beach (I know. I'm very fancy). This plan would also be great for getting you into shape for any other big event – like a wedding!

Six weeks out

With six weeks to go until your holiday, you have a great timeframe to get in fantastic shape. And, most importantly, you have enough time to do it sensibly and not do any silly crash diets. It's important at this stage that you take control of your eating and there are some nutrition tips to help with this on page 150.

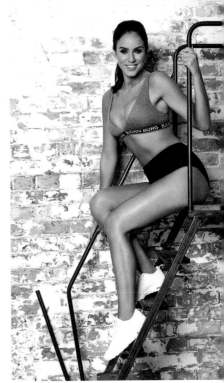

The first step is to take measurements and pictures of where you are now. People always hate this bit, as they're often so unhappy with how they look they'd rather not know the measurements. But trust me, in six weeks when you can see the difference in the pictures and on the tape measure, you'll be glad you did (and you can show all your mates).

Another good reason to do this is because you see yourself all the time, so you're unlikely to notice the changes to your body and it's easy to become demotivated. The pictures and measurements will provide reassurance that you're moving in the right direction.

You'll be training four times a week, doing three gym workouts and then one other workout of your choice. Let's get started.

Safety notice! If you're unsure how to use any of the machines, ask a member of staff at the gym for assistance. Don't be shy – they're there to help.

This is your training schedule for the next two weeks:

Six weeks out					
Monday	Tuesday	Wednesday	Thursday	Friday	Saturday or Sunday
Workout 1	Workout 2	Rest	Workout 1	Rest	Workout 2 or your choice of workout

Here is what your workouts will look like:

Workout 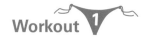 1

Five minute warm-up cardio of your choice. I like to use the bike or rowing machine.

For every exercise listed below, it's a good idea to do 1–2 warm-up sets with some lighter weights. This will get your muscles warm and also give you an idea of the right weight to use for the given number of reps. Remember, it's always better to start light and build up.

A1: Leg Press 4x12 reps

This is to work your thigh muscles. Sit in the machine and place your feet in position, shoulder-width apart. Slowly lower, bending your knees and then push the weight back up. Don't lock out your knees; always keep a slight bend in your legs to keep the muscle working and prevent injury.

A2: Bent-Over Dumbbell Rows 4x12 reps

This is to work your back muscles. Holding some dumbbells with your arms straight, bend over as if you are bowing, slightly bend your knees; your upper body should be parallel with the floor. Hold that position, keeping your back straight and pull the dumbbells towards your body, keeping your elbows tucked into your body, then slowly lower back down.

Go straight from the leg press into your rows and then rest for 60 seconds. Repeat four times before moving on to the B exercises.

B1: Leg Curl 4x12 reps

This is to work your hamstrings (the backs of your legs). Lie flat on the machine, with your ankles under the pad, shoulder-width apart. Keeping your hips pressed into the pad, curl your ankles up towards your bum, pause there and slowly lower.

B2: Push Ups 4x12 reps

These are great for your chest, shoulders and arms. Place your hands on the floor, shoulder-width apart, directly under your shoulders. Either lift up onto your toes or your knees – this is your start position with your arms straight. From here bend your elbows and imagine squeezing your shoulder blades together as you lower, pause just shy of the floor and push back up.

Do both of these exercises (B1–B2) in a row before resting for 60 seconds. Repeat four times before moving on to the C exercises.

C1: Dumbbell Biceps Curl 3x15 reps

Holding two light dumbbells, either stand or sit with your shoulders back and arms hanging down. From here bend your elbows and lift the dumbbells up towards your shoulders, squeeze your arm muscles and slowly lower.

C2: Dumbbell Lying Triceps Extensions 3x15 reps

Take a hold of two dumbbells – probably the same weight as the ones you used for your biceps curls. Lie on your back on a bench with your arms straight up in the air and from here carefully lower back towards your shoulders, then pause and lift back up. Keep them in line with your shoulders to avoid your face!

C3: Ball Crunch 3x15 reps

Sit on a stability ball with your feet shoulder-width apart. Slowly walk your feet forwards and lie back on the ball so it's supporting your lower back. From here squeeze your stomach muscles and crunch up 45 degrees, pause and slowly lower back down.

Do all three of these exercises in a row (C1–C3) before resting for 40 seconds. Repeat this three times.

Five minute cool-down cardio (I use the bike) and gentle stretching.

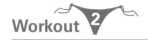
Workout **2**

Five minute warm-up cardio of your choice.

A1: Dumbbell Lunges 4x12 reps each leg

Holding a dumbbell in each hand down by your side, step forwards with one leg and slowly lower your other leg towards the floor, push through your front leg back to the start position, then do the same with your other leg.

A2: Dumbbell Standing Shoulder Press 4x12 reps

Standing, lift up a dumbbell in each hand so they are in line with your ears with your palms facing forwards. From here lift them up and bring them together above your head, then slowly lower back down to where you started.

Go straight from the lunges into your shoulder press and then rest for 60 seconds. Repeat four times before moving on to the B exercises.

B1: Dumbbell Squat 4x12 reps

Holding a dumbbell in each hand by your side with your arms straight, feet shoulder-width apart, bend your knees and push your hips back as if you were sitting down. Lower until your thighs are parallel with the floor and, pushing through your heels, come back up. You can actually sit on a chair or bench if you are struggling with this.

B2: Lat Pull-Down 4x12 reps

Take a hold of the bar on the pull-down machine, just outside of shoulder-width, and sit down with your knees under the pad. Pull the bar down to level with your chin using your back muscles and then slowly raise back up.

Do both these exercises (B1–B2) in a row before resting for 60 seconds. Repeat four times before moving on to the C exercises.

C1: Dumbbell Lateral Raise 3x15 reps

Either standing or seated, hold a light dumbbell in each hand down by your side with your arms straight. Keeping your arms straight, lift them out to the side and up to shoulder height, pause and slowly lower back down.

C2: Front Plank 3x20 seconds

These are brilliant for your core. Lie down with your forearms on the mat and your elbows under your shoulders. Either lift up from your toes or knees and hold your body straight. There should be a straight line from your shoulders to your knees or feet. Pulling your belly button towards your spine, hold that position.

C3: Side Plank 3x20 seconds each side

This time lie on your side with just one forearm on the floor, lift your body up from either your toes or knees. Again, there should be a straight line from your shoulders to your knees or feet. Hold that position.

Do all three of these exercises in a row (C1–C3) before resting for 40 seconds. Repeat three times.

Five minutes cool-down cardio and gentle stretching.

For your three weekly gym sessions, simply alternate between these two workouts. You'll see that for every pair of exercises in these programmes, it will require one piece of equipment, as well as either dumbbells or body weight. This is to make it easier for you in the gym. You can take dumbbells over to the machine and switch easily from one workout to another. In a busy gym, if you're moving from machine to machine there's a good chance someone will jump on in between and disrupt your momentum. This way you can almost reserve the machine until you've finished all your sets.

For your fourth session of the week, you can either repeat one of these workouts or do something of your own choosing. You could attend a class, go swimming, go for a long walk or jog. You do whatever works for you, providing it's for at least 45 minutes and gets your heart rate up.

Follow this routine for the first two weeks then we'll be stepping things up.

Four weeks out

Right, it's four weeks until your holiday. If you've been following the programme from the start you should have two weeks of hard training and good eating in the bank. If you haven't, don't worry. There's still time.

I want you to take your measurements and pictures again to see how you're getting on. If you know that a few nights out or pizza binges have held you back, now is the time to knuckle down.

For the next two weeks you're going to train five days a week doing four gym workouts and then a fifth workout of your choice. For your fifth workout of the week, you can either repeat one of the gym workouts or do something of your own choosing, as above.

These will be the same workouts as the last two weeks, but to step things up we are going to add 10 minutes of HIIT cardio on to the end.

When you're doing your resistance exercises it's important that you continue to challenge yourself. They should never feel easy. You'll begin to get a better idea of the weights you use for each, but you should be constantly trying to increase these. Push yourself! No pain, no gain and all that.

As well as these workouts you should be aiming to be as active as possible in your everyday life.

This is your training schedule for the next two weeks:

Four weeks out					
Monday	Tuesday	Wednesday	Thursday	Friday	Saturday or Sunday
Workout 1	Workout 2	Rest	Workout 1	Workout 2	Your choice of workout

Here are your workouts:

Workout 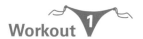 1

Five minute warm-up cardio of your choice.

A1: Leg Press 4x12 reps

A2: Bent-Over Dumbbell Rows 4x12 reps

Go straight from the leg press into your rows and then rest for 60 seconds. Repeat four times before moving on to B exercises.

B1: Leg Curl 4x12 reps

B2: Push Ups 4x12 reps

Again, do both these exercises in a row before resting for 60 seconds. Repeat four times before moving on to C exercises.

C1: Dumbbell Biceps Curl 3x15 reps

C2: Dumbbell Lying Triceps Extensions 3x15 reps

C3: Ball Crunch 3x15 reps

Do all three of these exercises in a row (C1–C3) before resting for 40 seconds. Repeat three times.

Ten minutes HIIT of cardio of your choice – I like to use the rowing machine or cross-trainer.

For your HIIT we are going to blast out 15 seconds as fast as you can, followed by 45 seconds nice and slow. Repeat ten times.

Five minute cool-down cardio and gentle stretching.

Workout 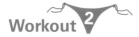 2

Five minutes warm-up cardio of your choice.

A1: Dumbbell Lunges 4x12 reps

A2: Dumbbell Standing Shoulder Press 4x12 reps

Go straight from the lunges into your shoulder press and then rest for 60 seconds. Repeat four times before moving on to the B exercises.

B1: Dumbbell Squat 4x12 reps

B2: Lat Pull-Down 4x12 reps

Again, do both of these exercises in a row before resting for 60 seconds. Repeat four times before moving on to the C exercises.

C1: Dumbbell Lateral Raise 3x15 reps

C2: Front Plank 3x20 secs

C3: Side Plank 3x20 secs each side

Do all three of these exercises in a row (C1–C3) before resting for 40 seconds. Repeat 3 times.

Ten minutes HIIT cardio of your choice.

For your HIIT we are going to blast out 15 seconds as fast as you can, followed by 45 seconds nice and slow. Repeat ten times.

Five minute cool-down cardio and gentle stretching.

Now it's time to ramp things up for the next week . . .

Two weeks out

It's only two weeks until you jet off to that sunny beach and if you've been working hard from the start you should be making great progress by now.

For those of you just starting, you need absolute focus on the goal here. You've got two weeks to get beach ready! I want you to take your measurements and pictures again at this stage. This will motivate you to see a real difference when we take them again in two weeks.

We're really stepping things up, so you're still doing four gym sessions this week, but with a twist. We're going to keep the same pairs of exercises in your workouts but we're now adding in 30 seconds of a high intensity exercise onto each one. For example, you'll do the leg press into dumbbell rows and then 30 seconds of burpees. It's tough! We're going to keep the HIIT cardio at the end too, but just for five minutes.

I also want you to do fasted cardio three days a week, ideally a 40-minute power walk (cardio performed on an empty stomach can help accelerate fat loss). Just get up, neck a black coffee and get walking. Other options would be walking on a slight incline on a treadmill, a swim, or 40 minutes on the cross-trainer or bike.

Here's your workout schedule for the next week:

Two weeks out			
Monday morning	Monday afternoon	Tuesday morning	Wednesday morning
40-minute power walk	Workout 1	Workout 2	40-minute power walk
Thursday afternoon	Friday morning	Friday afternoon	Saturday or Sunday
Workout 1	40-minute power walk	Workout 2	Your choice of workout, rest on the other day

And here are your workouts:

Workout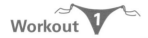

Five minute warm-up cardio of your choice.

A1: Leg Press 4x12 reps
A2: Bent-Over Dumbbell Rows 4x12 reps
A3: Burpees 4x30 secs

Get in position as if you were doing a push up, from here bend your legs and jump them forwards so your knees are in line with your hands, then stand up and jump in the air. Place your hands back on the floor, jump your feet back to the start position. That's one burpee.

Complete all three exercises (A1–A3) then rest for 60 seconds. Repeat this four times then move on to the B exercises.

B1: Leg Curl 4x12 reps
B2: Push Ups 4x12 reps
B3: Squat Thrusts 4x30 secs

These are like the first part of the burpee. Start in a press-up position, and from here bend your legs and jump them forwards so your knees are in line with your hands. Then jump them back so your legs are straight again. That's one squat thrust.

Complete all three exercises (B1–B3) then rest for 60 seconds. Repeat four times then move on to the C exercises.

C1: Dumbbell Biceps Curl 3x15 reps
C2: Dumbbell Lying Triceps Extensions 3x15 reps
C3: Ball Crunch 3x15 reps
C4: Reverse Lunges 3x30 secs

Reverse lunges are very similar to dumbbell lunges, except you step backwards and aren't holding any weight. Standing with your feet shoulder-width apart, step backwards with one leg, lowering your knee towards the floor. Push back up to the start position and repeat on the other leg.

Complete all four exercises (C1–C4) then rest for 60 seconds. Repeat three times then move on to the HIIT cardio.

Five minute HIIT cardio of your choice.

For your HIIT we are going to blast out 15 seconds as fast as you can, followed by 45 seconds nice and slow. Repeat five times.

Five minute cool-down cardio and gentle stretching.

Workout 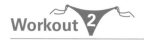 **2**

Five minute warm-up cardio of your choice.

A1: Dumbbell Lunges 4x12 reps

A2: Dumbbell Standing Shoulder Press 4x12 reps

A3: Jump Squats 4x30 secs

Jump squats are like your dumbbell squats except you are jumping up and not holding any dumbbells. As with your dumbbell squat, stand feet shoulder-width apart, bend your knees and push your hips back, slowly lower then push through your heels and jump into the air, bend your legs as you land and repeat.

Complete all three (A1–A3) exercises then rest for 60 seconds. Repeat four times then move on to the B exercises.

B1: Dumbbell Squat 4x12 reps

B2: Lat Pull-Down 4x12 reps

B3: Squat Thrusts 4x30 secs

Complete all three exercises (B1–B3) then rest for 60 seconds. Repeat this four times then move onto the C exercises.

C1: Dumbbell Lateral Raise 3x15 reps

C2: Front Plank 3x20 secs

C3: Side Plank 3x20 secs each side

C4: Bench Step-Ups 3x30 secs

Complete all four exercises (C1–C4) then rest for 60 seconds. Repeat three times then move on to the HIIT cardio.

Five minute HIIT cardio of your choice.

For your HIIT we are going to blast out 15 seconds as fast as you can, followed by 45 seconds nice and slow. Repeat five times.

Five minute cool-down cardio and gentle stretching.

In addition to your fasted cardio and gym workouts, I want you getting super active wherever possible. If you start to feel faint in workouts or lacking in energy you may need to increase your carbs slightly. It's important that you have enough food so that you can train hard and recover from the sessions. Cars can't run on fumes and neither can you. You need to fuel all this training.

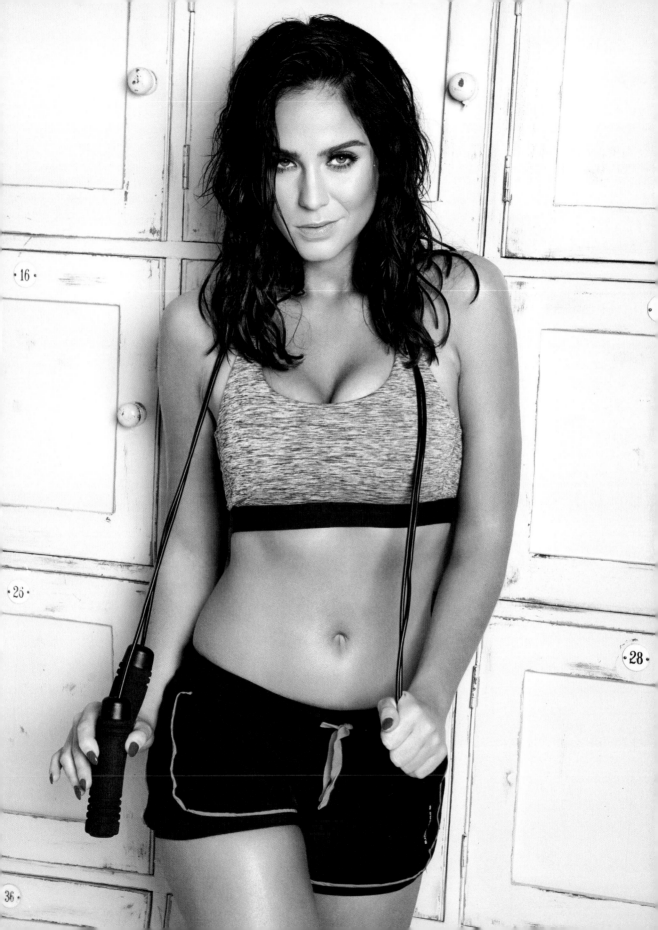

One week out

One week to get that beach body! Whether you've been following from the start or you've left it late, you can still make some significant progress in a week. Especially with the week I've got planned for you.

The programme is the same as last week's but this time you are doing 45 seconds on your high-intensity exercises rather than 30. I also want you to go for a 40-minute fasted power walk on five of the next seven days. As well as that, you'll be doing five days' training in the gym. That's ten sessions in the next week!

Here's your schedule:

One week out				
Monday morning	Monday afternoon	Tuesday morning	Tuesday afternoon	Thursday morning
40-minute power walk	Workout 1	40-minute power walk	Workout 2	40-minute power walk
Thursday afternoon	Friday morning	Friday afternoon	Saturday morning	Sunday afternoon
Workout 1	40-minute power walk	Workout 2	40-minute power walk	Your choice of workout

Here are your workouts:

Workout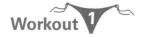

Five minute warm-up cardio of your choice.

A1: Leg Press 4x12 reps

A2: Dumbbell Row 4x12 reps

A3: Burpees 4x45 secs

Complete all three exercises (A1–A3) then rest for 60 seconds. Repeat this four times then move on to the B exercises.

B1: Leg Curl 4x12 reps

B2: Push Ups 4x12 reps

B3: Squat Thrusts 4x45 secs

Complete all three exercises (B1–B3) then rest for 60 seconds. Repeat this four times then move on to the C exercises.

C1: Dumbbell Biceps Curl 3x15 reps

C2: Dumbbell Lying Triceps Extensions 3x15 reps

C3: Ball Crunch 3x15 reps

C4: Reverse Lunges 3x45 secs

Complete all four exercises (C1–C4) then rest for 60 seconds. Repeat this three times then move on to the HIIT cardio.

Five minutes HIIT cardio of your choice.

For your HIIT we are going to blast out 15 seconds as fast as you can, followed by 45 seconds nice and slow. Repeat this five times.

Five minute cool-down cardio and gentle stretching.

Workout 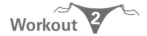 2

Five minute warm-up cardio of your choice.

A1: Dumbbell Lunges 4x12 reps

A2: Dumbbell Shoulder Press 4x12 reps

A3: Jump Squats 4x45 secs

Complete all three exercises (A1–A3) then rest for 60 seconds. Repeat this four times then move on to the B exercises.

B1: Dumbbell Squat 4x12 reps

B2: Lat Pull-Down 4x12 reps

B3: Squat Thrusts 4x45secs

Complete all three exercises (B1–B3) then rest for 60 seconds. Repeat this four times then move on to the C exercises.

C1: Dumbbell Lateral Raise 3x15 reps

C2: Front Plank 3x20 secs

C3: Side Plank 3x20 secs each side

C4: Bench Step-Ups 3x45 secs

Complete all four exercises (C1–C4) then rest for 60 seconds. Repeat this three times then move onto the HIIT cardio.

Five minutes HIIT cardio of your choice.

For your HIIT we are going to blast out 15 seconds as fast as you can, followed by 45 seconds nice and slow. Repeat this five times.

Five minute cool-down cardio and gentle stretching.

Congratulations!

You smashed it. Now's the time to take a final photo and compare it to the original – I guarantee you'll notice a difference. Enjoy your holiday knowing you've really achieved something and are in great shape.

And if you didn't manage the full six weeks . . . or any of the programme at all . . . rock that bikini anyway. I bet you look gorgeous!

Some amazing pre-holiday nutrition pointers. Because it's not all about the gym

Choose your carbohydrates wisely!

Carbohydrates don't have to be the enemy, but the type that you choose is important. As a general rule, go for complex carbohydrates over refined ones. For example, have brown rice instead of white.

Sugar is the most refined carbohydrate and too much in your diet can hinder your weight-loss goals. Keep an eye on food labels – as a general rule, anything over 15 grams of sugar per 100 grams is classified as a high-sugar product.

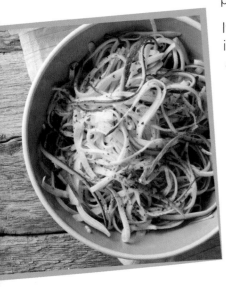

If you are looking to reduce your overall carbohydrate intake, you could try using non-starchy vegetable alternatives such as cauliflower mash, (see page 181) instead of mashed potato, or courgette 'pasta' (using a spiraliser) instead of wheat pasta.

Keeping blood sugar levels stable is a key factor in avoiding energy slumps when you might be tempted to go for a biscuit or sweets to pick you up. Combining complex carbohydrates with protein and healthy fats is a good way to help lessen the overall blood-sugar impact of a snack or meal. For instance, eating an apple with a small handful of walnuts.

Don't neglect your post-workout nutrition! The hour after your workout – often referred to as the 'anabolic window' – is not just for body builders. During this time, the muscles you've been putting to work are most receptive to nutrients and need the amino acids (found in proteins) to help them repair and recover. A protein supplement alongside some simple, refined carbohydrates (yes, this is the time that you do want a bit of a sugar boost!) can help to drive the amino acids into the muscles to help them recover. This will help you get toned and bikini ready!

Eat clean wherever you can. It goes without saying that if you make it from scratch, you know what's going into your food. That's not always possible if you're busy, so if you do buy processed food check the labels for natural ingredients and be very wary of anything labelled as 'reduced fat'.

Keep hydrated! You should aim to drink 6 – 8 glasses of water a day, but how much you need can depend on temperature and how much you are sweating it out in the gym.

The holiday clothes I can't be without

This dress screams Grecian goddess to me.

I think when you've got a tan light colours really pop; creams and whites are gorgeous in the summer.

I also love long, floaty stuff. You have to accept the fact that if you're in a hotter climate you're going to be sweaty and you want to be comfortable. I love embracing maxi dresses and clothes with long chiffon layers.

It's nice to make an effort to look glam on holiday, but you can do it in a more low maintenance, laid-back way. This dress can be worn with a pair of heels and gold jewellery for a night out, or you can whack it over the top of a bikini and wear it with flip-flops. I think it's important to pack clothes that can be multi-purpose.

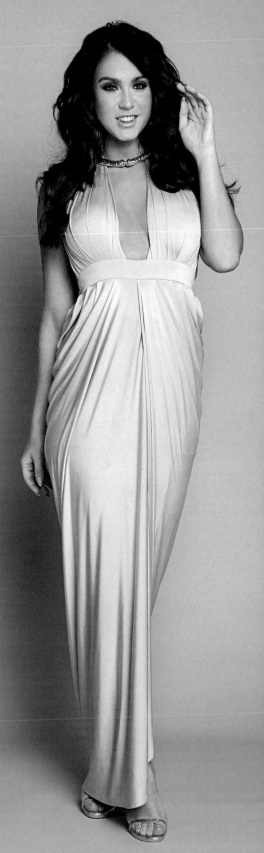

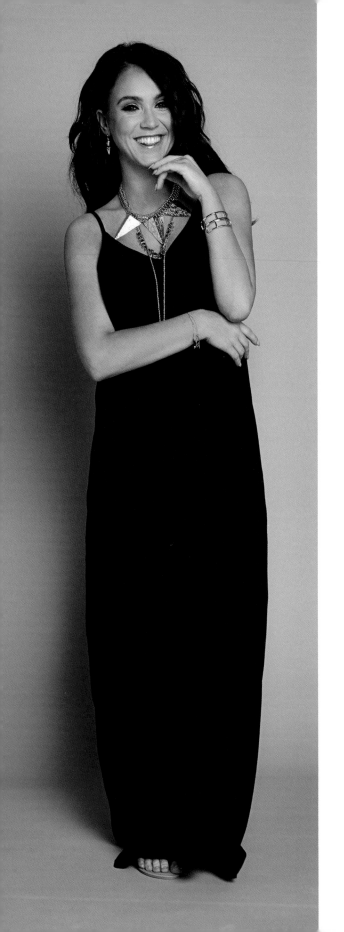

Don't be afraid of wearing black on holiday. A lot of people shy away from it and think their holiday wardrobe should be only bright or white, but black can look really sexy – and every good holiday wardrobe has to include a couple of maxis.

The beauty of black is that it gives you a blank canvas so you can let your accessories do the talking. You could even whack a long-line cardi over this dress and wear it to travel home in because it's so comfortable.

This yellow number can be dressed up or down and it's lovely for a night out – it would be perfect for sundowners. It's sexy without being over the top.

Bright colours are a must for holidays and you may as well make the most of being able to get away with wearing crazier shades. I can't imagine myself strolling down Newcastle High Street in a bright yellow dress like this, but it really suits a sunny place. Luckily I have the same dress in loads of different shades, including black! (If you find a style you love, which suits you and makes you feel really confident, get it in every colour!) Yellows, oranges and mint green are great for summer.

Floral, Aztec patterns and broad horizontal stripes are lovely on holiday. These trousers are so comfortable because they're wide-legged and flared. This whole look is smart and chic without being too try-hard. It's definitely a bit different too and it's nice to branch out. You've got your legs covered but you've got your abs and your shoulders out, so it's still quite sexy.

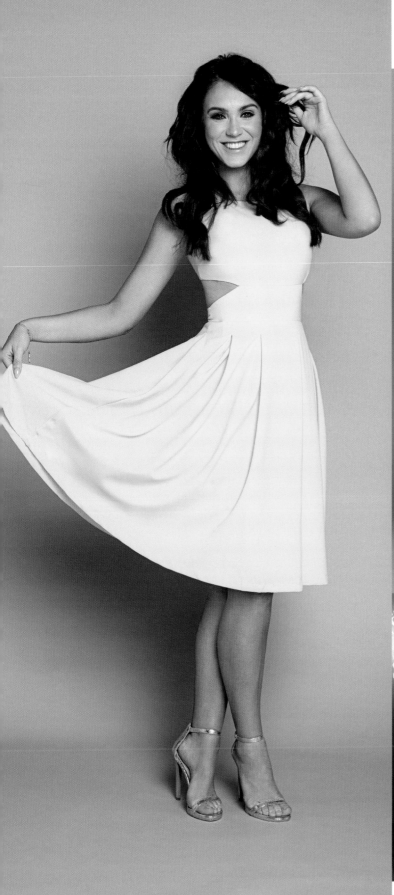

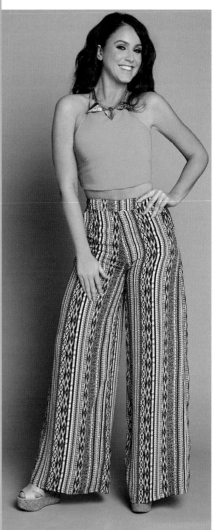

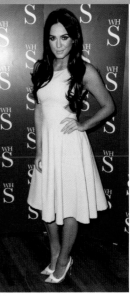

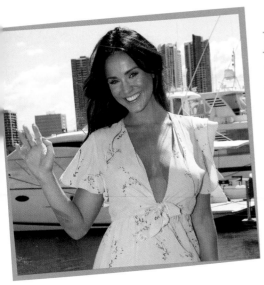

Don't wait until your holiday to get a tan

Something I would recommend people do before they jet off is to get a spray tan. Not only will you be able to wear all your lovely summer clothes from day one and feel confident, but you also won't look like Casper's sister on the beach.

There's this myth that if you have a fake tan you can't get a real tan, but that's absolutely not true. However, fake tans don't have UV protection so make sure you apply plenty of high-factor sun cream at all times.

My tanning guidelines

It's no secret that I love a little bit of fake tan. Well, a lot. I swear by spray tans, and Fake Bake is my favourite. They do every shade and option going – it's the best!

✳ I always exfoliate and shave before I get a tan to make sure I've got all of the old fake tan off.

✳ Don't have a hot shower before you apply any kind of fake tan, because you open your pores and you'll get dark spots on your skin.

✳ San Tropez Self Tan Bronzing Mousse is very good if you've got the luxury of time. If you're going out on a Saturday you can apply it on a Friday night with a mitt, shower in the morning and you're good to go with a nice natural colour.

✳ If you're pushed for time, Fake Bake's 5 Minute Mousse Self-Tan develops almost instantly. Those are both what I like to call 'stay on' fake tans because they won't wash off as soon as you have a shower.

✳ If you've left tanning until the last minute or you're having an impromptu night out, don't panic. Get yourself some Rimmel Instant Tan Sun Shimmer, which gives you a sun-kissed glow in minutes. You can get it in matte or shimmer, and the shimmer is great for a night out. It's got more coverage and because it's sparkly you feel like you're properly going for it.

✳ Be warned that if you cry or it rains it could come off though, and no one wants to look like a zebra when they're out on the pull.

I always use this thing called a Bronzie when I fake tan now. It's a godsend. I used to get fake tan all over my clothes and sheets, and I'd also have white patches on my skin where I'd rubbed my fake tan off by mistake. Every time I did my own fake tan at home, I used to have to pad around my house like a damp, darkened mess for ages until it dried. Now I swear by these onesies that you can wear over the top of your freshly applied tan.

They're made of breathable material with a zip all the way down. And there are ventilation holes in the places you sweat, like under your arms. They also lock in that biscuity smell that blokes hate! I quite often go and get a spray tan and then bomb about the shops in my Bronzie afterwards. I'm not ashamed.

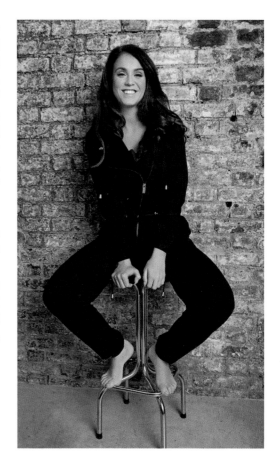

Get beachy waves, whether you've been to the beach or not

* There are two different ways to get beachy hair, but both start with you rough-drying your hair – this means using your hairdryer and fingers to dry the hair, keeping any natural waves intact.

* You can then tong the hair to create waves – but make sure you don't curl the ends! Form a tight spiral around the tong but leave the ends out so they stay straighter.

* The other way to do it is to curl your hair around your straighteners and twist them round to create a kink.

* Loosen the waves using your fingers and finish with a salt spray. It dehydrates the hair, and hair naturally tries to bend when it's dehydrated so it will give it a good texture and shape.

Holiday make-up

You don't want to pile on the make-up on holiday when you've got a natural glow, but if you can't bear to go completely bare here are some sun-friendly suggestions.

✳ Waterproof eye-pencils are great for holiday. **Urban Decay** do a range called **24/7** that really last; **GOSH Forever Eye Shadow Pencils** are a great cheap-and-cheerful alternative.

✳ I would also suggest having semi-permanent lashes done before you go away because they'll make you look like you're wearing mascara at all times. I had these done pre-jungle and it made all the difference.

✳ It's really important to use make-up with an SPF in it. BB creams are great – **Bobbi Brown**'s contains SFP 35 and **Maybelline's Dream Fresh BB** is SPF 30, so there's no need to layer sun lotion on top of either.

✳ You can also get lip tints and glosses with SPFs in them. **MAC** do a good **Tinted Lip Conditioner** that's SPF 15 or you could try **No7's BB Lips** with SPF 15.

✳ You don't need bronzer when you've got a tan, so I use a highlighting stick to give my skin a shimmer instead. **NARS The Multiple** is a great multi-purpose highlighting stick in a range of colours, that can be used for eyes, cheeks, lips and body! Perfect for when you want to travel light. **The Collection Speedy Highlighter** is a good affordable alternative.

I hate packing, but I'm pretty good at it now

Packing is the bane of my life because I do it so often, but as a result I've got it down to a fine art.

I always used to over-pack and take 24 bikinis for two weeks, and I'd always end up wearing the ones I liked best over and over.

We all have a tendency to take too much when we go on holiday and you end up coming home with a case half full of clean clothes. So don't put clothes in because you think you *might* wear them. You're better off just taking things you love and washing them while you're out there so you can wear them more than once.

If in doubt, you can always write out a plan of what you want to wear every day so you know exactly what you need. You don't have to stick to it 100 per cent, but at least that way you'll know you've got enough clothes to last you.

Less is more when it comes to holiday packing. You basically need three or four bikinis and loads of comfy sundresses. I also take one big beach bag, one over-the shoulder handbag for going out, and then a couple of really nice outfits in case you're going for a meal or a sunset cruise. Throw in a beach towel and a load of suntan lotion and you're done.

When it comes to shoes I normally take one good pair of sandals for going out, a nice pair of wedges and a ton of flip-flops. I don't think you have to spend a fortune on flip-flops either. I'll buy them from anywhere. Occasionally I'll treat myself to a pair from Kurt Geiger, but they'll be proper leather with loads of jewels that will last me all summer. Don't bother to invest a lot in something you're just going to wear around the pool. Flip-flops are going to get dirty and they're going to break, and if they were £3 from the market no one's going to be crying over their sangria if they snap in half. And you can also chuck them away at the end of the holiday so there's more room for shot glasses and bottles of Absinthe for your mates.

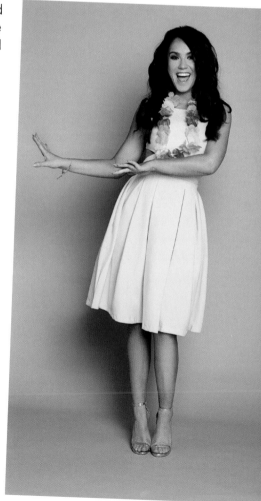

Some other good packing tips I've learnt are:

✳ Stick to a maximum of five colours so you can mix and match everything you take.

✳ Put tumble dryer sheets at the bottom of your case to keep your clothes smelling fresh.

✳ Put a cotton wool pad in your pressed face powder to prevent it breaking.

✳ Wrap cling film or masking tape around the lids of liquids so they don't spill.

✳ Pack your underwear in your shoes. Why waste all that space?

✳ Roll all of your clothes. They'll crease less and seem to take up less room.

✳ Keep your make-up brushes safe by storing them in an old sunglasses case.

✳ Stack your bras on top of each other so they keep their shape.

HOW TO MEND A BROKEN HEART

It involves chocolate and Adele . . .

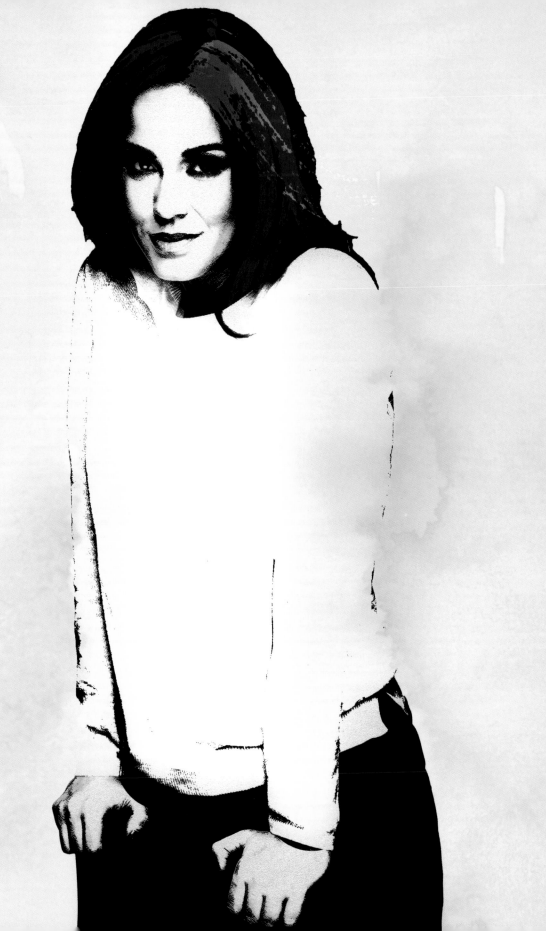

Break-ups suck. The end.

I don't know a single person who hasn't *been through a horrible break-up at some point, and I firmly believe that the best way to get over someone is to get under someone else.*

I don't mean you should to go out and jump into bed with someone or use them as rebound fodder, but why not have some fun and go on some nice dates? What have you got to lose?

After a break-up you can cry for days, go out and get plastered with your mates for weeks on end, or you can go and sit with monks in Tibet and reflect on your relationship. You can join a gym, get a new haircut, buy a load of new clothes, and all of those things may help. But ultimately the only way you can truly get over the person who broke your heart is when you get together with the next person. Simple as that.

Don't rush into it if you don't feel ready, but that is the one thing that truly helps you to move on. I always think about my exes until I start seeing someone else. I think that's just how the mind – and the heart – works.

The important thing to bear in mind when you're throwing yourself on the floor and sobbing is that it's okay to still be upset about your ex days, weeks, months or even *years* after you split up. (But hopefully *not* years.) There is no time limit on feeling crap. Whether you were together for five minutes or five years, you need to grieve and mourn that relationship.

Lads and lasses deal with break-ups in totally different ways. So don't worry about how your ex is handling it, because the chances are whatever he does will annoy you.

This is usually how it works:

Month 1

* A girl will generally spend the first month after a split crying her eyes out.

* Her ex will be out partying.

Month 2

* The girl will be starting to get her life back together.

* The lad is hungover and tired and reflecting on whether he's made a mistake.

Month 3

* The girl has got a new lad and she's happy.

* The lad is in a right mess.

That's because girls grieve and get clarity. Girls get their confidence back and then they go out and meet someone else when they're ready. But guys don't deal with it properly. They just go out and get drunk and don't talk to their mates, so all the issues are unaddressed and they suffer later. That's happened to me so many times with exes.

Thanks to social media we see everything these days, and lads will often put up posts showing what a great time they're having. When you're cut-up and heartbroken and all you see is them having a good time, you don't look past it and see that most of the time it's bravado. It makes you feel like you didn't mean anything to them.

Break-ups make you feel so confused. One minute you want to block the lad's number, and the next you want to Facetime them non-stop or turn up at their door. You go through all these different stages and the thing is, there's no magic trick for getting through it. The only thing you can do is surround yourself with your friends and do things to take your mind off it. And if you want to cry, cry.

There's no time limit on how long it takes you to get over a lad. I've got mates who will break up with someone one weekend and be out on the lash with us girls and necking on with someone else the following one. But I've also got friends who broke up with lads back in the nineties and they're still not over it. People get over things in different ways and you've just got to find out what works best for you.

When I break up with someone, I do try to be respectful and mindful of their feelings, because I know what it feels like when someone else moves on quickly. I surround myself with my friends and do things that were difficult to do when I was in the relationship, like go out with all my lad mates.

I go shopping and buy myself into something new. I go to the gym and I focus on *me.* Doing things that took a back seat when you were in a relationship is a great idea. Quite often you'll have ditched your gym sessions for nights in on the sofa eating pizza, and when you look in the mirror you still see the person you were when you were with that guy. It can be difficult to shake off the memory of him.

If that is the case, give your image a shake-up so the person who looks back at you in the mirror isn't the heartbroken girl she was; she's a sassy, confident woman who's ready to take on the world and book a holiday to Magaluf with the lasses.

I'm one of those girls who likes to flirt with other lads and get attention if I'm feeling a bit vulnerable or unwanted. But if I do that, I'm keeping it casual because the chances are I won't be emotionally ready to have another relationship – even if I feel like I am.

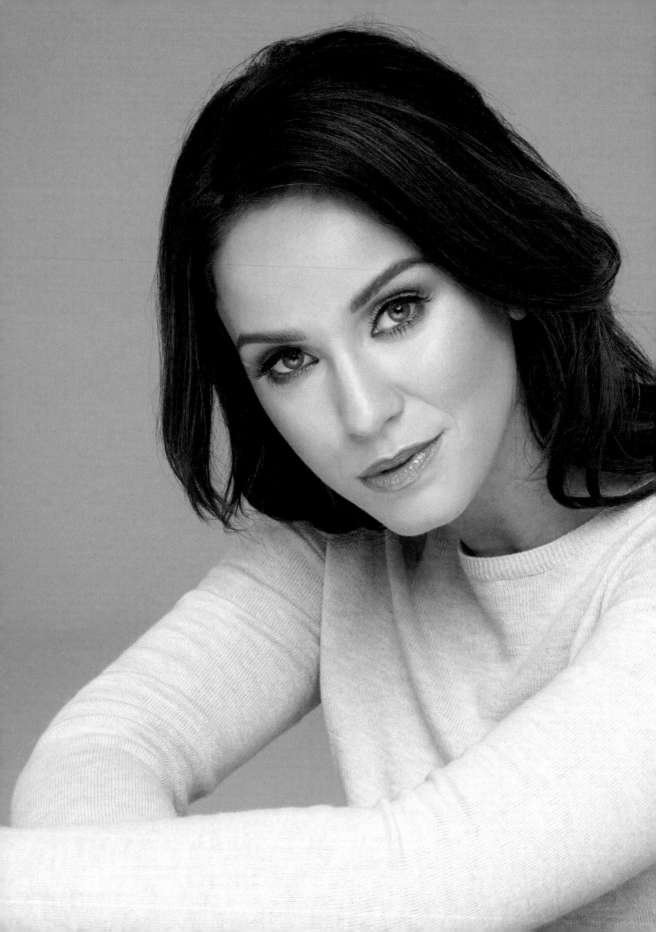

There's a temptation to go out and start seeing someone else so you feel that same closeness but it's just not the same, so take it with a pinch of salt and have fun. Go on dates and tash on with fellas, but don't leap into something big for the sake of it.

Company and time are the main things that will get you through. There's a lot to be said for getting drunk with your girl mates and having a good cry when you need to. It doesn't matter who finished with who. Even if you made the decision, there will always be that feeling of loss. Don't be afraid to be emotional. There is no such thing as over the top when you're going through a break-up. Allow yourself a bit of self-pitying and wallowing. Whack *Bridget Jones* on, get a tub of Cookie Dough ice-cream and a bucket of wine and shout things at the telly. Slag him off, get angry and get it all out.

My worst break-ups

Delightful Dean

I've been through quite a few break-ups and I have been quite unlucky in love over the years. Or maybe all those lads were unlucky because they couldn't pin me down? And I was lucky because I escaped from some proper knobs? My first ever break-up from my boyfriend Dean was one of the hardest. First loves are always the best, and don't let anyone tell you any different. Your true love will be the most amazing *ever,* but your first love will be a close second and that's because it's all new and it's exciting. It's like your first drink of the night: you can chase that buzz for the rest of the evening but nothing will be quite as good.

The difficult thing with Dean and me was that neither of us did anything wrong. There was no great cheating saga or argument; we just slowly grew apart. I wanted to go to Magaluf for the summer and then go to uni in Liverpool, and Dean wanted to stay in Newcastle and be a joiner. Staying in Newcastle and settling down just didn't factor into my plans at that point, and unfortunately that meant I had to make a pretty grown-up decision to break up with him. It would have been impossible to keep things going when I was moving away.

It was so confusing because I knew Dean was great for me, but I wanted to live my life. I was only 17 and I think because we didn't have any kind of big dramatic bust-up, we kept gravitating back to each other and falling in and out of the relationship. We didn't seem to be able to cut ties altogether and that made things so

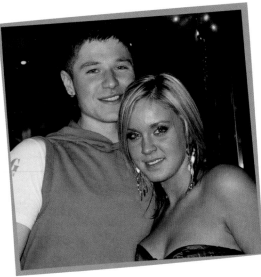

Vicky 4 Dean!

much worse. In the end we decided to make a complete break, but I did still wonder if we should be together.

Then he got a new girlfriend and suddenly the decision was taken away from me. Until that point I always kind of felt like the ball was in my court. It wasn't something I played on, but it was something I was aware of. Then all of a sudden I didn't have the control any more because he was dead happy with someone else. It hurt so much to see him doing everything he used to do with me with this new girl, but at the end of the day it had been my decision to break up and he had every right to move on and be happy.

After that, it was a case of pulling my socks up and telling myself I'd made the right decision. Doing the season in Magaluf helped loads because it meant I got away and had a proper break. I was working and partying so hard I didn't have time to obsess over him.

Dean and his new girlfriend eventually broke up and we've met up loads of times over the years. We still get on really well and it's lovely. It just goes to show that we made the right decision by splitting up when we did, because we've managed to salvage a pretty nice friendship.

Tricky Ricci

The most high-profile split I've ever had was with Ricci Guarnaccio. There will always be lads you look back on and think, *Why did I ever let them go?* Then there will be those lads you look back on and think, *What the hell was wrong with me? Why did none of my mates tell me I was dating such a bellend?* And for me, that lad is Ricci.

The relationship was so toxic. It hurt while I was in it, and it hurt even more when I was out of it. If you've read my autobiography you'll know all the details about our relationship, and maybe you've had a similar one yourself at some point. Ricci was controlling and I couldn't live my life the way I wanted to. After we finally broke up, Ricci kept telling me he couldn't live without me and begging me to get back with him – I felt so guilty. But I also knew he had an agenda. It's horrible when someone tells you their life is nothing without you, but the relationship wasn't right and I never really trusted his motives.

I think everyone assumed that because I'd been the one to call time on the relationship, I'd be happy and ready to move on, but I wasn't. I was getting over the break-up of an engagement and I was really hurting. Even though the relationship is bad you still have to live with that big hole in your life and there are times when you miss the company.

> ## Then there will be those lads you look back on and think, *What the hell was wrong with me? Why did none of my mates tell me I was dating such a bellend?* And for me, that lad is Ricci.

The way I got over Ricci was by focusing on myself, getting into training in a big way and cracking on with my career. I gave my life a real sense of purpose and I found myself again after being one half of 'Vicky and Ricci' for so long. For a long time I hadn't had a solo identity, but I found this crazy sense of clarity from putting myself first. And the stronger I got physically, the stronger I got mentally; I realised I could cope with anything. Once you get out of a bad relationship and focus on yourself, you have the opportunity finally to figure out what you're made of. And that's exactly what I did.

Un-Bear-able

Another break-up that had a big impact on me was my split with Stephen Bear, which is weird considering it was a drop in the ocean compared to some of my other relationships. We were only together for about six months, but it burn really brightly for that short amount of time. Looking back, I wasn't in love, but I was mad for him and we were very obsessed with each other. I loved his company and we essentially almost lived together.

It was tough to get over him because I didn't *want* to. I didn't want to finish with him and that's why it was so hard. I knew he wasn't right for me and I knew he'd cheated and only really cared about himself, but I still fell for him in a big way.

The hardest thing for me to face up to was the fact that I been willing to let myself be treated like that. It was a big wake-up call when I realised he was walking all over me and I was the only one who couldn't see it. Everyone was telling me I shouldn't be with him and I was about to lose everything, including the respect of best mates and my family.

We kept splitting up and getting back together which is such a slippery slope; it's much better to just make a clean break. In the end I did call time on our relationship once and for all.

I remember sitting down with some of my lad mates not long after we had broken up and crying about all the rumours I'd heard about Bear with other women. They said to me: 'You know what this looks like, Vicky? Classic playground behaviour. He's a boy who's trying to get a girl's attention, but he's hurt and this is the way he's dealing with it.'

Getting a lad's perspective really helped because obviously I think like a girl, and once I realised what he was doing it made things easier.

I strapped on my lady balls, took a deep breath and focused on work again. I did a big book tour, shot a massive ad campaign for my clothing collection and made some brilliant videos for my website. I also saw people I hadn't seen for a while because I'd been distracted with Bear, and I did things that made me happy and gave me a boost. Even small things like buying a really nice new lipstick helped.

I told myself repeatedly that I was okay and I didn't miss Bear, and as the weeks passed I realised I wasn't pretending any more. I wasn't *telling* myself I was okay any more – I *was* okay.

I strapped on my lady balls, took a deep breath and focused on work again.

Songs to blare out after a break-up

For the immediate post-break-up crying-and-snot-fest stage

* *Someone Like You* by Adele

* *Listen* by Beyoncé

* *I Will Always Love You* by Whitney Houston

For the angry-drunk-singing stage

* *I Knew You Were Trouble* by Taylor Swift

* *Love The Way You Lie* by Eminem featuring Rihanna

* *Rolling in the Deep* by Adele

* *If I Was a Boy* by Beyoncé

* *Cry Me a River* by Justin Timberlake

For the screw-you-I'm-over-you stage

* *I Don't Care* by Cheryl Cole

* *Irreplaceable* by Beyoncé

* *Zero* by Chris Brown

* *All I Do Is Win* by DJ Khaled

* And of course . . . *We Are Never Ever Getting Back Together* by Taylor Swift

Basically, if you put Taylor Swift, Adele and Beyoncé on rotation, you can't go wrong!

Break-up brownies (*makes about 16*)

Sadness needs food, and that food is chocolate. Dry your tears and make these amazing double-chocolate brownies.

Ingredients

175g plain chocolate, broken into chunks

200g butter, cut into pieces, plus extra for greasing

4 large eggs

325g caster sugar

100g self-raising flour

50g cocoa powder

150g white chocolate, broken into chunks

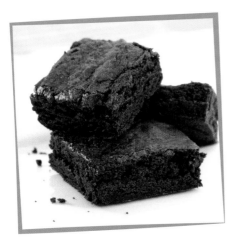

Method

1. Preheat the oven to 180° C. Grease the sides and line the bottom of a 23cm baking tin with baking paper.

2. Put the chocolate and butter in a heatproof bowl. Pour about 2cm of hot water into a small saucepan and sit the bowl on top, but don't let the bottom of the bowl touch the water. Set the pan over a low heat, stirring occasionally, until the chocolate and butter have melted. Leave to cool slightly. (Or you can cover the bowl with cling film and microwave on high until melted.)

3. Crack the eggs into a mixing bowl and add the sugar, then whisk using an electric mixer for 3 minutes or until thick, pale and creamy. Pour the melted chocolate mixture into the bowl and gently stir it in so you don't lose any air.

4. Put the flour and cocoa powder into a sieve, and holding it over the brownie mixture, tap the sieve until the flour mixture is sifted into the bowl. Gently mix it in until everything is combined, then stir in the white chocolate.

5. Tip the mixture into the prepared tin and gently spread it out into an even layer. Put the tin in the oven and bake for 25–30 minutes until the edges start to come away from the sides of the tin but the centre is still slightly soft. (Don't forget the best bit, licking the bowl!) Leave the brownie to cool completely in the tin, and then turn it out onto a wire rack. Cut the brownie into 16 squares– and eat them all.

How to clear your head, boost endorphins and get you feeling like you again

Training can be an amazing way of clearing your head and making you feel better when everything feels pretty crappy. When you're blasting through a really tough training session, you don't have time to think about some bellend who broke your heart. You can totally lose yourself in the workout.

Training is *your* time away from the stresses of the day, and it's also a great way for you to feel like you are getting back some control in your life. You can train hard and feel good about yourself again on *your* terms. Your body naturally produces chemicals called endorphins in response to pain or extreme exertion, and that's why you often come away feeling on such a high after a great workout.

A really tough spin class with a banging soundtrack is ideal. You can push yourself really hard without worrying about hurting yourself. Another good option is a boxing session, which I love because you can take out your anger and aggression on those pads.

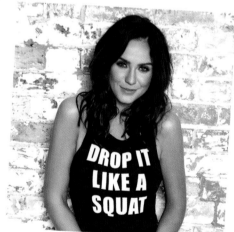

Music can be brilliant for psyching you up to train hard too. Put together a playlist of your favourite or most motivational songs (this is where Beyoncé comes in again) and destroy that workout. Music can also encourage your body to produce more endorphins so combining music and exercise is a break-up win-win.

A DAY IN THE LIFE

Workin' 9 to 5 with Vicky Pattison.

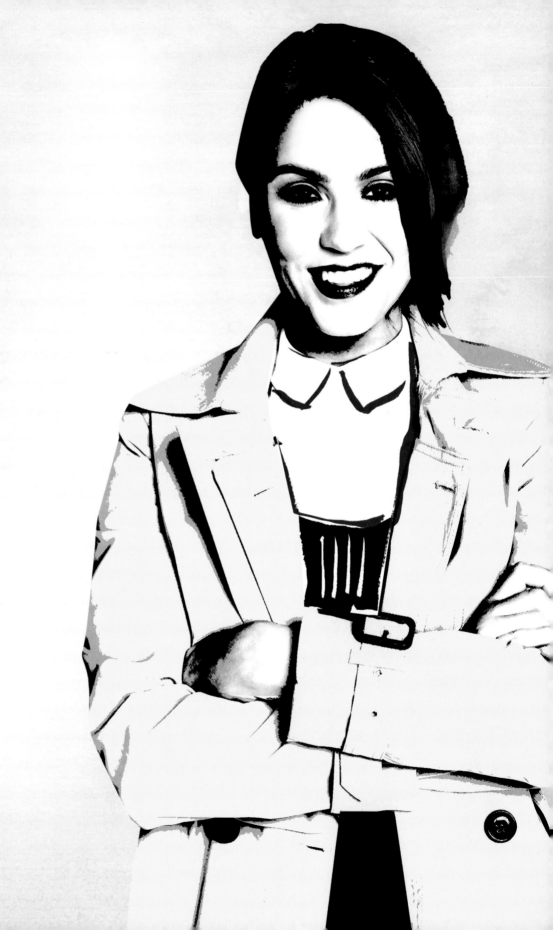

A day in the life of Miss Vicky Pattison

(I can't stand it when people talk about themselves in the third person!)

I don't really have a typical day, because it's rare for any two days to be the same for me – unless I go back to Newcastle for the weekend, when I tend to follow more of a pattern: see my friends and family, go shopping, get drunk, laze as much as possible.

I keep my own diary and my agents also have one for me, so ridiculously I know what I'm supposed to be doing a year from now, but I don't always know what I'm doing tomorrow. My schedule changes so often I can never be sure that what's meant to happen will actually happen when it's supposed to.

I'm totally fine with that though because as I've mentioned before, I've never wanted to be in a nine-to-five job because I get bored really easily.

My morning skincare routine

The first thing I do when I get up is cleanse my face. I'm a big fan of Rodial skin products and I cleanse with their Super Acids X-treme Exfoliating Glycolic Cleanser. Then I like to moisturise with the Dragon's Blood Sculpting Gel Serum, which can honestly make me look like I've had an extra eight hours in bed . . . always handy if I've been out the night before.

Breakfast

If I'm at home I'll have Scott's oats with semi-skimmed milk and blueberries and raspberries on top. Or scrambled eggs on toast. If you're going to be sassy you can add avocado, chorizo and chilli. Or a spinach and mushroom omelette is great. If you're in a rush, little porridge pots, yoghurt or my Mini V shakes can be grabbed on the run.

This morning I had yoghurt, fruit and nuts and a green tea. I avoided carbs for reasons you will find out later!

Breakfast yoghurt mix (*serves 1*)

Ingredients

125g organic, live, natural yoghurt

1 nectarine (chopped)

1 tablespoon hemp seeds

1 tablespoon chopped Brazil nuts

Method

Mix the ingredients together and serve!

Benefits: *The combination of protein and healthy fats from the nuts and seeds in this will help to keep you full during the course of the morning.*

Live, natural yoghurt contains friendly (probiotic) bacteria which are needed for healthy digestion and immunity.

Brazil nuts are also packed with selenium. This mineral is a really important antioxidant used in the body to help combat free radicals.

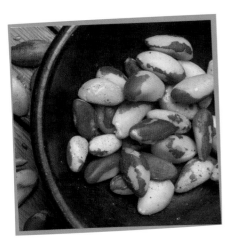

Why I always try to go to the gym in the morning

I love going to the gym first thing, and I'll always do that if I'm not due to be on telly early. I get my headphones on and just go. Because I'm working out on an empty stomach I'm burning fat rather than the calories I've just eaten.

I tend to train in the morning because (a) it's when I can fit it in most easily, and (b) it sets me up and puts me in a good frame of mind.

Quite often, if I book in a training session or plan to go later in the day, a meeting come up with takes precedence and I have to cancel, which drives me mad. The good thing is that not many people want to have meetings at 7 a.m., so if I go then I'm usually pretty safe!

My workout routine can be really changeable because I'm travelling so much. Sometimes I'll end up working out in a hotel room or the hotel gym, and sometimes I manage to get some one-on-one time with a personal trainer, which is my favourite thing to do.

When I'm back home I always work with a guy called Robbie Thompson, who I've known for years. He helped me get into shape after I'd let myself go due to drinking a year's worth of calories every time I filmed *Geordie Shore*.

Robbie totally turned things around for me at a time when I wondered if I'd ever get back to feeling like myself again. My bum was down by my knees and my whole body shook every time I waved at someone. Something had to be done.

I would recommend everyone to get a trainer when they first start out on a fitness journey, or if they're going back to the gym after a long time away. I know it's expensive but even if it's only for a couple of sessions, they can set up a good programme for you and get you on the right track. It's no good strolling along a treadmill for ten minutes and then going for a sauna when you go to the gym, and that's what you could end up doing if you don't get any proper direction.

Personal-training sessions will give you a routine early on, and you won't let yourself cancel those appointments because they'll cost you money.

If you're not feeling very flush why not find a training buddy and either get a trainer between you or work out together? Schedule the gym in your diary just like you would a work meeting or a doctor's appointment and tell yourself you can't miss it just because you don't fancy it. At the end of the day, you wouldn't just not turn up to an important meeting because you can't be bothered, so why do the same at the gym?

Getting a personal trainer changed my life for the better, and that's not just me being dramatic. Getting back in shape gave me confidence and drive, and a lot of that was down to Robbie pushing me. If you feel strong, you feel like you can do anything, and working out gives you that extra push you need.

Exercise was my saviour when everything in my life felt pretty rubbish, and to this day it's my go-to pick-me-up when things get tough. It clears my mind

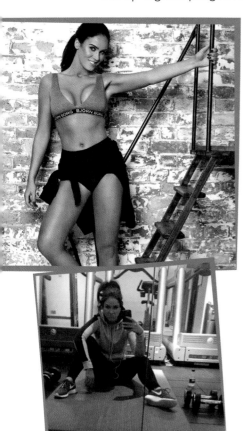

Gym fantasy vs gym reality.

and that time I have in the gym, my hotel room or even in a park, is *my* time – and that makes it really special.

Looking after yourself isn't self-indulgent – it should be second nature. There's nothing quite like that feeling of accomplishment when you know you've worked really hard in a session and your body is going to be working well for the rest of the day.

I've always wanted to look strong as well as lean, and actually *be* fit, not just look it. It's easy to bulk up in the gym and look really muscly, but underneath your body may be a mess. I like to train every part of myself. I hate it when I see guys with a really massive upper body and tiny legs. I just don't get that.

My training now is a combination of heavy lifting on things like deadlifts and squats, higher rep compound exercises on movements like lunges and rows, and then high intensity, lung-busting exercises like prowler pushes, bike and rowing machine intervals. The variation means my routines are fun and I don't get bored. I'm constantly working different parts of my body and trying new things, and it's something I'll carry on doing for the rest of my life.

This is one of my favourite morning workouts

A1: Trap Bar Deadlift 4x15 reps

Holding either a normal bar or trap bar, with your hands shoulder-width apart, start at the bottom position of a squat. Keeping your back straight, push through the floor and push your hips forwards to strand up with the weight. Push your hips back and slowly lower back towards the floor, again keeping your back straight.

B1: Back Squat 3x5 reps

This is the same as a bodyweight or dumbbell squat (see page 140) except this time you have the bar on your shoulders, with your hands on the bar just outside of your shoulders. Stand with your feet shoulder-width apart, bend your knees and push your hips back as if you were sitting down. Lower until your thighs are parallel with the floor and, pushing through your heels, come back up. Again, you can sit onto a chair or bench if you are struggling with this.

B2: Leg Press 3x15 reps (See page 138.)
B3: Leg Extensions 3x25 reps

Sit upright in the machine, with the pad on your shins. Squeezing your thigh muscles, lift the pad up until your legs are straight, pause and slowly lower back down.

C1: Dumbbell RDLs* 3x12 reps

Stand up straight with your feet shoulder-width apart, holding two dumbbells in front of you, resting on your legs. Slightly bend your knees, push your hips backwards and at the same time bow your upper body down, keeping your back straight. As you do this, keep the dumbbells against your legs and lower them to around your knee; you'll feel a stretch in the back of your legs. Squeeze your bum muscles and push your hips forwards to stand back up.

*RDL = Romanian Deadlift!

D1: Lat Pull-Downs 3x12 (See page 140.)

D2: Dumbbell Shoulder Presses 3x12 reps

Seated upright, lift two dumbbells up so they are in line with your ears with your palms facing forwards. From here, lift them up and bring them together above your head, then slowly lower back down to where you started.

E1: Dumbbell Triceps Extensions 2x15 reps

Take a hold of two dumbbells, probably the same weight as for your biceps curls. Lie on your back on a bench with your arms straight up in the air, from here carefully lower back towards your shoulders, pause and lift back up. Keep them in line with your shoulders to avoid your face!

E2: Dumbbell Lateral Raises 2x15 reps

Either standing or seated, hold two light dumbbells down by your side with your arms straight. Keeping your arms straight, lift them out to the side and up to shoulder height, pause and slowly lower back down.

F1: Prowler Sprints 5x20 secs with 40 secs rest

The prowler is basically a sledge with handles that you push along in front of you, like a bobsleigh! Get into a sprinter position with your back straight, holding the prowler, and sprint as fast as you can for 20 seconds.

The intensity of the exercises means I burn plenty of calories in the session, and my body will continue to burn them long after I've finished my workout.

If I do stay in a hotel that doesn't have a gym and there isn't one nearby, I'll usually do a HIIT-style workout in my room using one of the routines I've talked about page 79, because I don't need any equipment for those.

I would always rather go to a gym to help me get in the right frame of mind, but if I'm working hard and putting in the effort I'm happy anywhere.

Fancy a nose inside my handbag?
Go on then . . .

My Prada bag was something I bought myself as a
congratulations present after I won the jungle.

I'd always wanted a classic Prada bag and this has been such an incredible investment because it goes with anything. I didn't have a boyfriend at the time so I knew no one else was going to buy it for me, and I thought I deserved a nice gift. Self-gifting is essential in my book.

The Prada purse was a gift from my lovely agents Gemma and Nadia, because they were so sick of me constantly scrabbling around for my bank card and having money floating around the bottom of my bag. It contains my cards, usually a hotel room key and some money and receipts. I love it and I use it to death. There's usually a pass to my publisher's office floating around in the bottom of my bag somewhere; I go to work there a lot – everyone in the building knows me by now!

I always keep make-up in my handbag because I never know how long my days are going to be or where they're going to take me. I have a face powder or bronzer, an eyeshadow palette and a contouring palette, mascara and a bit of lip gloss and lip balm. That's all I need really.

I have headphones in case I want to listen to music, and they're so good if I'm travelling somewhere by train because I can completely switch off.

I usually have a couple of little bits and bobs of jewellery in my bag in case I end up going out on the lash and I want to accessorise an outfit. And an emergency bottle of fake tan!

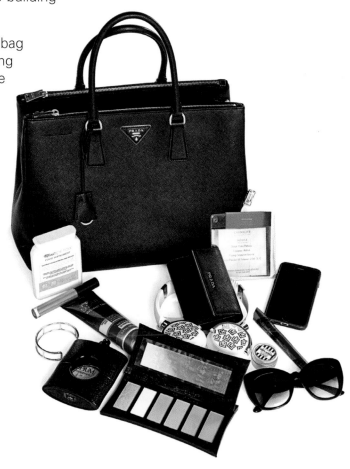

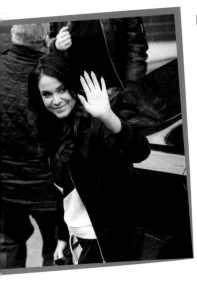

I always have sunglasses in my bag for obvious reasons, and I've learnt the hard way to put them in a proper box and not in one of those silly cloth bags, because otherwise they get scratched or broken.

My mam is never without a hand cream and now I'm following in her footsteps and I always have one.

I always have some Mini V necessities, like a shake in case I don't get a chance to have breakfast or I have to work through lunch. Mini V Fat Burners give you energy if you're having a long day, and the Mini Detox are for when you're feeling like a bag of piss with a hangover. If you have two with some water after a night out and then two the following morning they'll help you to feel bright eyed and bushy tailed.

I like strong perfumes that last all day and Opium by YSL is one of my favourites. I also love Decadence by Marc Jacobs, Flowerbomb by Viktor and Rolf and Ghost by Calvin Klein. I'm never without perfume in my handbag.

Today is a busy day . . .

I managed to get a workout in first thing this morning, which is always a huge bonus. I didn't have any TV commitments but I did have a photoshoot to get to, because I had to do some promo shots for a campaign.

My call time was 10 a.m., and a car picked me up from my hotel in Waterloo at nine, so I had plenty of time to get to the studio in East London. The traffic in London is notoriously bad if you're travelling at the wrong time so I always like to have buffer time.

When I arrived on the shoot I went straight into hair and make-up. Depending on how glammed-up I need to be, that can take anywhere from an hour to two hours.

I was working with hair stylist Chloe Oakes and make-up artist Krystal Dawn, who I've worked with a lot and I just love them. We got to have a good catch-up and a gossip, and I also spent a lot of time on my phone doing work and looking at social media. (And, I'm not going to lie, I had a little nap too.)

Having my hair and make-up done is one of my favourite thing about shoots. The bit I don't like is having the actual pictures taken. I'm not that confident in front of a camera and I never will be. People are often surprised when I tell them that but it's my least favourite part of the job generally, which is why

I always try and work with photographers that put me at ease.

Because my days are so unpredictable I can't often plan what I'm going to eat, but I made sure I drank loads of water from the moment I got to the shoot.

I don't believe in cutting out carbs at all, but sometimes they can make you bloat a bit so I avoid them when I'm doing a shoot, hence I skipped the wholemeal toast at breakfast time.

For lunch I had a big chicken salad with loads of rocket, peppers, sundried tomatoes and cucumber with a balsamic and olive oil dressing. I also had a Diet Coke, which is one of my big vices. I know they're not great but I don't overdo them. They're more of an 'every now and again' treat.

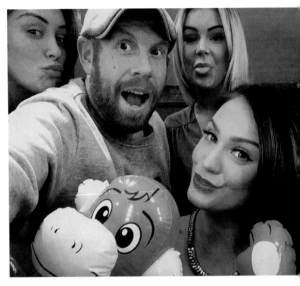

Here I am with my glam squad for this book, make-up artist Krystal, photographer James and hair stylist Chloe. And a photobombing monkey.

It's party time!

When the shoot finished, I got myself dressed to go out that night and called a cab. I'd been invited to a clothing launch and some of my friends were going along, so we arranged to meet up first.

Because I'd already had my hair and make-up done that saved me loads of time, and there was no point in going back to my hotel first. I arrived at the shoot wearing leather trousers, an oversized shirt and some boots, so I've swapped the boots for heels, added some jewellery and I was good to go.

I had a protein bar in the taxi into central London so I didn't get hungry and eat unhealthy canapés at the party, and after a couple of drinks my mates and I headed to the RaRa Room in Piccadilly. I only had a couple of drinks because I was due on *This Morning* the next day and I didn't want any kind of hangover. I stuck to gin and slimline tonic because I do believe that the darker the spirits, the worse the hangover.

I was home relatively early but I had to grab something to eat on the way home, which isn't ideal. I don't really like eating late but sometimes I don't have any choice. I grabbed a Leon Superfood Salad Box, ate it back at the hotel and I was in bed by 11 p.m.

Goat's cheese and pomegranate salad (*serves 2*)

This is an amazing lunchtime salad recipe if you've got time to make something up yourself . . . like I never do!

Ingredients

100g goat's cheese (crumbled)

3 handfuls of rocket (roughly chopped)

3 spring onions (chopped)

150g cherry tomatoes (halved)

1 red pepper (chopped)

1 handful of walnuts (chopped)

70g pomegranate seeds

For the dressing

4 tablespoons pomegranate juice

2 tablespoons hemp oil (or olive oil)

1 tablespoons lemon juice

Method

1. Mix the salad ingredients together.

2. Mix the dressing ingredients together.

3. Add the dressing to the salad just before serving.

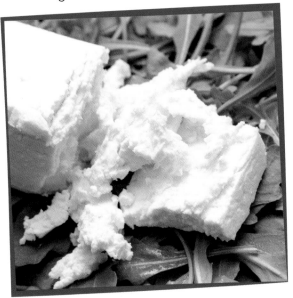

Benefits: *Pomegranate adds some sweetness to the salad, giving an antioxidant boost and walnuts contain omega 3 essential fatty acids.*

Red pepper and tomatoes are both good sources of vitamin C for a healthy immune system.

Rocket is a bitter (but tasty!) salad vegetable that support digestion and detoxification.

Lemon and ginger salmon with cauliflower mash (*serves 2*)

What I would have eaten for dinner, if I'd been at home . . .

Ingredients

2 x Salmon fillets

1 dash of lemon juice

1 large pinch of cayenne pepper

1 teaspoon chopped ginger (this can be bought prepared and frozen)

1 garlic clove (crushed)

2 teaspoons chopped parsley (this can be bought prepared and frozen)

For the cauliflower mash
(makes 4 portions)

½ medium cauliflower

1 garlic clove (crushed)

1 tablespoon coconut oil

On the side

1 handful of green beans (chopped)

Method

1. Preheat the grill to a medium heat and place the salmon fillets on a grill pan (skin side down).

2. Squeeze the lemon juice over the fillets and sprinkle the cayenne pepper over them.

3. Mix the ginger, garlic and parsley in a small ramekin or bowl then rub the mixture evenly into the flesh of the salmon.

4. Grill the fillets for 10 minutes or until cooked through.

5. Meanwhile steam the cauliflower florets and the green beans. Once the cauliflower is soft (when tested with a fork), transfer to a bowl. Add the garlic and coconut oil and mash or purée until smooth.

6. Serve each salmon fillet with half of the cauliflower mash and half of the green beans.

Benefits: *Salmon is a great source of protein and omega 3 essential fatty acids, which help to control inflammation in the body, and support healthy skin.*

Cauliflower mash is a low carbohydrate alternative to mashed potato that tastes much better than you'd think! Garlic adds flavour and gives your immune system a boost.

Can I go to sleep now?

I feel like I've had a really productive day. I got a good training session in, I did some work, caught up with friends and my diet was bang on. I had a couple of drinks, but life is for living, isn't it?

Before I got into bed I brushed my teeth, washed my face and threw my clothes on the floor (sorry). I'm not the world's best at remembering to take off my make-up properly, but do as I say not as I do: take your make-up off properly! I had a glass of water before bed and two Mini V Detox tablets because sometimes a sneaky couple of drinks can get you when you least expect it. They can creep up on you without your realising and that's the last thing you need when you're going on live TV the next morning!

Sometimes I really struggle with sleeping, and I've tried all sorts of things to combat that over the years. I always stop drinking caffeine at around 4 or 5 p.m., and that includes green tea and Diet Coke. I'm not a coffee drinker and I don't smoke, so I don't have to worry about those. I would definitely recommend cutting out all caffeine if you find sleeping tricky.

I always keep a notepad by my bed because I often start thinking about things late at night and it feels like impossible to get them out of my head unless I write them down. Or I'll need to remember something in the morning and I'll get anxious that I won't. Writing things down makes me feel much calmer.

You should also endeavour to stop looking at your phone a good hour before you go to sleep because the light stimulates your mind. If you absolutely have to use it, turn the brightness right down.

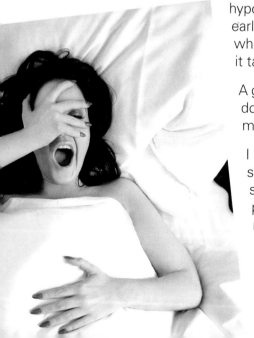

I'm one of the worst for that so I don't want to sound hypocritical, but I am teaching myself to put it down earlier and earlier. And try not to look at social media when you're in bed. One annoying comment can be all it takes to keep you awake for hours.

A good book helps me to chill out and wind down. But don't read anything too dramatic or it may get your mind racing again.

I think ultimately having a day that has left you satisfied and fulfilled is the best way to guarantee sleep. If I know I've exercised, eaten right and been productive that helps me to drift off and I wake up ready for the next day.

My favourite books

To Kill a Mockingbird, Harper Lee

I really like the message of the book. I love that this one bloke is striving to teach these kids right from wrong in a society that is so ignorant and corrupt.

American Sniper, Chris Kyle

It's a very sad but powerful story.

The Hunger Games, Suzanne Collins

I love escapism and as soon as you start reading the *Hunger Games* trilogy you can't put the books down.

All the **Harry Potter** books, J. K. Rowling

I will forever be upset that I'm not a wizard. I must have read the full series of books three times. They're so captivating.

Tom Clancy's **Jack Ryan** novels.

Tom Clancy is a really clever writer and his books really hold my attention.

Autobiographies

I also love autobiographies and it will come as no surprise that I loved Cheryl Cole's. Simon Cowell's unofficial one was great too. That's where I learnt about Simon's ability to remember everyone's name, and that's why I always try and do the same. You can pick up so much information about your idols from reading autobiographies and I love getting that insight.

And anything I've written, obviously!

THE CONFIDENCE TRICK

Fake it till you make it . . . everyone else is!

11

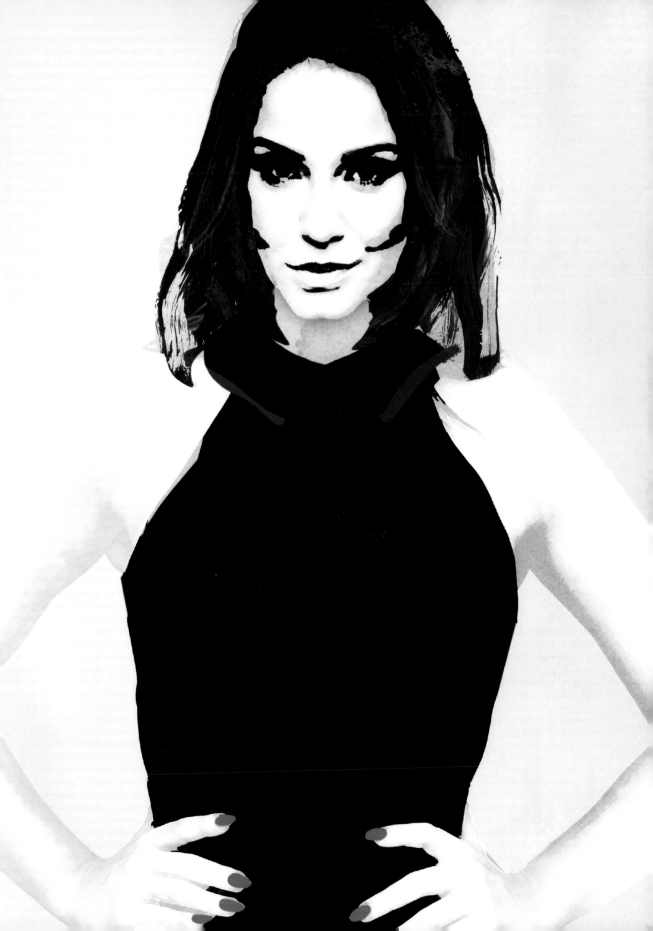

Confidence is a funny thing

Confidence is a tough one, because it can come and go – and you can feel much more confident in some situations than others. And sometimes it can be hard to anticipate which situations are going to be the ones that will cause you to have a wobble.

People think I'm really confident, but like anyone I've joked and laughed through situations but been agonising over things inside.

I went on a weekend away to Monaco and I was so nervous because I was going with a group of very posh people. (Yes, it was with Spencer. I'm sure you've seen the pictures!) I was talking to my mam about it before I went and she said to me: 'Don't you worry about it. Go and show everyone how to have fun.' I went, I was myself and I ended up having a brilliant time. I got on with everyone really well and I think that's because I just cracked on. I tried not to worry about anyone judging me and as a result I was able to relax and have a laugh.

Confidence comes from being yourself and being happy with who you are, and not worrying about what's going on in other people's lives or judging them. Loving the way you are and being confident is sexy. Looking down your nose at someone? Not sexy. And if any of those people had talked down to me it would have put me off them straight away. Thankfully they were secure enough in themselves not to feel the need to do that.

> **Humans aren't meant to be perfect. You're meant to be unique and have flaws, and that's what makes you amazing.**

In some ways, I'm definitely more confident than I was when I was younger . . . but in others I'm not. My sister always says I'm the most insecure I've ever been because I'm under constant scrutiny. The more well-known I've become, the more mindful I've had to be of everything I say and do. I used to do things with reckless abandon because I could. I didn't have anyone to answer to and the worst that could happen if I got thrown out of a bar for being mortal was that I'd have to apologise to a few people the following day. But now if Vicky Pattison from the telly does something like that it could be front page news, so I'm much more scared of making a mistake.

But when it comes to myself as a person, I feel happier with who I am than I ever have. I think that comes with age and accepting that you'll never be perfect. Humans aren't meant to be perfect. You're meant to be unique and have flaws, and that's what makes you amazing.

On a shallower level, a really nice outfit and getting my hair and make-up done can make me feel great in the moment. I'm never going to be a size zero, but dressing for my shape has given me confidence. Accepting that I don't, and never will, look like a Victoria's Secret model has made me much happier generally.

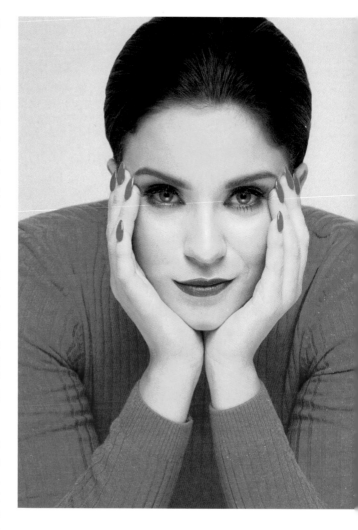

There are a lot of people in the world who judge you on how you look and dress. But none of that matters unless your personality shines through. People who are ugly inside *look* ugly. If you're nice to people and you've got something to offer in terms of a sense of humour or kindness, people will like you for it.

Always remember you're worth a lot and you bring something to the table, because *everyone* does. You've got special qualities so don't obsess about being like someone you see in a magazine because most of the time what you see isn't real.

For years I thought that in order to succeed you had to be stoic and aggressive. And that's actually completely untrue. Being confident and strong doesn't mean you have to be hard and cold. I'm so sensitive and I cry over anything, whether it's a TV advert or someone telling me a story, and I like that about myself. Being able to show your emotions is a sign of confidence. You're baring your soul and showing who you really are, and nothing is more attractive when you're getting to know someone. Emotions aren't a weakness.

Beauty is only skin deep and your worth isn't about how pretty you are. It's about how you treat and help other people. We rise by lifting others. If you're mean and you're bitter and you're jealous, people will see it straight away.

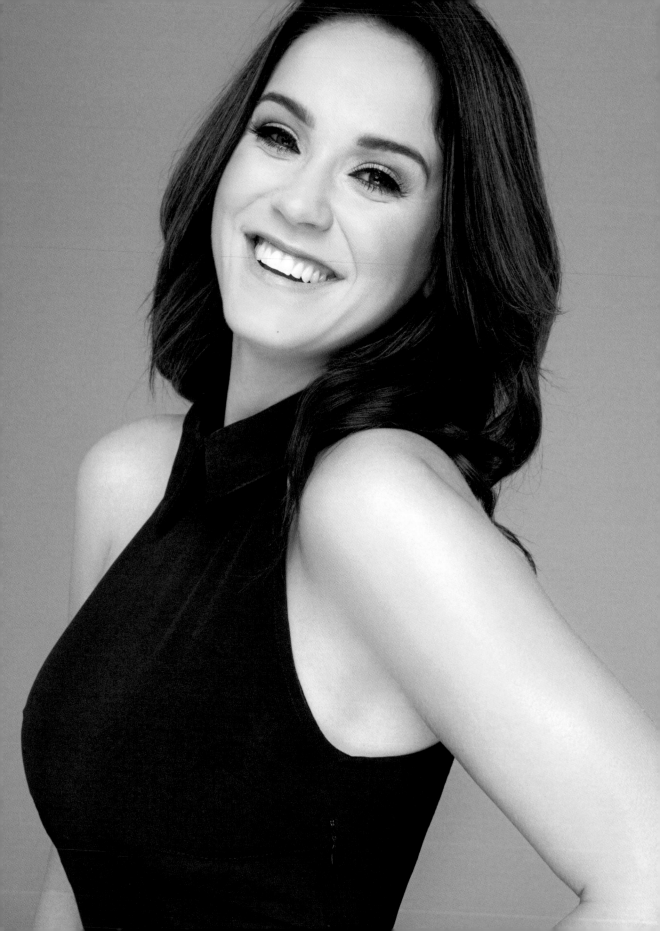

My rollercoaster weight-loss journey

Feeling good about yourself – not just the way you look, but feeling strong and healthy – is key to confidence. I've already talked a bit about how I lost weight with the help of my trainer Robbie Thompson and gained a much healthier attitude towards food. But as we all know, when you lose weight it isn't the end of the story.

The hardest thing for me now is keeping the weight off when I've got the busiest lifestyle I've ever had. My days can be 20 hours long and sometimes I have no time to train. I'll be in a studio with a massive plate of pastries, pre-made sandwiches and chocolate. And if I'm working late, sometimes Domino's is a quick, easy option.

I think every woman out there can identify with what I'm saying because we're all super busy, whether that's with our careers, our social lives, kids, relationships and family. It's tricky to balance being on the go all the time with being fit and healthy.

Food-wise, I snack on things like nuts and berries, and if I'm really up against it I find online food delivery services incredible. I promise I haven't changed and I don't spend loads of money having all my meals cooked for me, but sometimes it's just a matter of convenience. Places like Soulmate Food and Fuel Station will send you your food for three days and it's all nutritious and balanced.

If you're got a really big event you want to slim down for, they're great if you've got the money. I swear by them when I've been busy and want to eat healthily in the easiest way possible.

My weight has been a struggle at times, and I have fluctuated since I left the jungle. I think it's partly because I was so excited about eating all of the things I'd missed, and partly because my lifestyle became so erratic so quickly.

But I take steps to make sure my weight doesn't go above about nine-and-a-half stone, which is where I know I'm comfortable. I'm not a slave to the scales and I tend to go more by how my clothes feel, but I do weigh myself every now and again just to stay on track. The good thing is that I know I can lose the weight because I've done it before, and that makes it easier. When weight goes on I focus on getting back into shape again and I do.

I would never starve myself and be silly because I have a good knowledge of nutrition now, and I know what works and is healthy. Faddy diets, detoxes, missing meals, leaving food groups out of your diet – none of these things are long-term solutions.

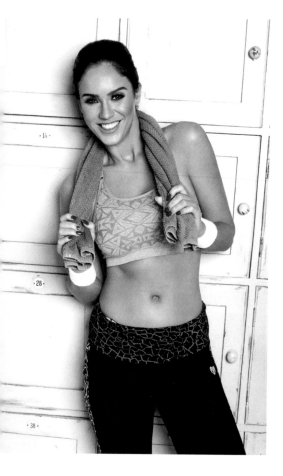

You shouldn't see a diet as something that's temporary. It's a lifestyle change so you've got to find what fits in best with your life and is doable. There's no point in going on a mad health kick for two weeks and then getting bored and going back to eating takeaways every night. You need balance.

I still drink, but I drink in a more civilised fashion. Whereas before I'd go out and binge drink, now I'll have a single drink at lunchtime if I've got a meeting, or I'll go out for dinner with my mates and have a few.

As I've said, what works for me is training first thing so my mind is already in a healthy place for the rest of the day. I feel like I owe it to myself to eat healthily after all the work I've done in the gym. I like to eat my slow-release carbs – like oats or brown bread – in the morning, and then I have protein-heavy meals with tuna, chicken or steak and loads of green vegetables for lunch and dinner. I drink a lot of water and green tea, and I do all of those things so that I can treat myself from time to time without feeling guilty.

Please don't think you have to live like a nun and train like a Trojan to be healthy. You don't. You need moderation and balance, and I'm discovering that more and more. I've also discovered that it's more difficult to lose weight as you get older, but I've got to take that one on the chin.

> **Please don't think you have to live like a nun and train like a Trojan to be healthy. You don't. You need moderation and balance, and I'm discovering that more and more.**

Don't be too hard on yourself because nutrition can fall by the wayside when you've got a lot going on and we all tend to fluctuate a bit. And sometimes a lot! But remember that you *can* get back to the weight you want to be. It may take a little while to do it sensibly but that's much better than panicking and doing faddy diets.

If you don't lose weight slowly and steadily you'll mess up your metabolism. Your body knows what you're doing and it will get mad at you. It will say, *I remember what you did last week when you starved me!* and it will hold on to the food you eat the following week for longer. Don't try and trick your body. It controls you, not the other way round.

Treat your body like a well-oiled machine. You have to clean machines, put good stuff into them and treat them with care if you want them to run smoothly. You can't neglect them. And it's the same for your body. If you put rubbish in your body it won't work properly. Eat well and take care of yourself and your body will find its natural weight, your skin will glow and you'll feel happier inside and out.

My main food rules

If you want to lose weight and get your body running smoothly it's all about the protein, so have loads of lean protein like salmon, prawns, skinless chicken breasts and good quality steaks. Ignore this whole thing about red meat being bad for you because it really doesn't hurt every now and again. And have loads of green veg like green beans, asparagus and broccoli. Pile your plate high with veg and then pick your carbs sensibly and have whole-wheat pasta, brown rice or sweet-potato mash. Avoid anything with sugar, if you can. Every refined food has loads it in and sugar is a toxin that sticks from your nipples to your knees.

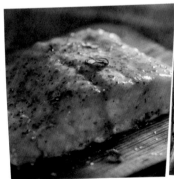 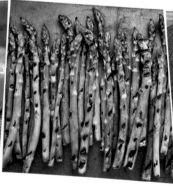 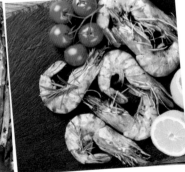

It's very hard for women to get their head around the fact that they have to eat *more* in order to lose weight. It took me a long time to realise that was true. You're going against anything you've been doing for years and it's so difficult to adopt a totally new way of thinking when you've been telling yourself you have to restrict the amount you eat for so long. Women tell themselves they need to eat less and do more cardio in order to lose weight and it's *so* wrong. You need to eat more of the right things and train with weights to get your body lean.

'Vicky Pattison fat' is a really popular Google search

If you type 'Vicky Pattison fat' into Google you get thousands of hits, and I think it's hilarious because it's who I was not who I am, and I'm not going to deny I was a bit too keen on biscuits for a while. But it's not always easy to bat off nasty comments.

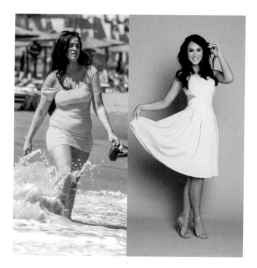

Criticism is a hard one because the way you deal with it totally depends on the mood you're in. If someone writes something nasty about me I can be very benevolent and try and understand why they did it. If I'm feeling good, I'll tell myself that it says more about them than it does about me. But if you catch me on a day when I'm down and tired and missing my family I can get really angry and upset about exactly the same comment.

There are two types of criticism: constructive and destructive. But both can be tricky to handle and constructive criticism can be difficult if someone remarks on something you're sensitive or passionate about.

For instance, I really struggle to take advice from my mam about my books, even though I know she's only trying to help. You have to be a bit humble and take the higher ground, and it's taken me a long time to get to that point because I'm so fiery and reactive. If someone says something I don't like I can get very defensive, and I've had to learn to stay calm and try to see things from the other person's point of view.

Friends and family trying to help you out and giving you advice is fine if it's helpful because it comes from a good place. And although it's hard to admit, you don't always know best about everything. It's sometimes harder taking criticism from someone close to you because you want them to think everything you do is wonderful. But they're just looking out for you, so you have to take a deep breath and suck it up.

Genuine meanness is different, but you do have to tell yourself that if someone is being purposely unkind it often comes from a very unhappy place. I would never walk up to someone in the street and say 'What the hell are you wearing?' or tell someone they'd put on weight. It's socially unacceptable and mean. Anyone who's brought up with manners and a basic respect for other people should be able to gauge what is and isn't okay. But people don't seem to get that on social media.

People don't think about the fact that there's another human reading their tweet or Instagram comment. I'm sure they think that because you're in the public eye you don't have feelings, but it still hurts. No matter how successful and happy you are, words still sting. I wish people would be more mindful of that. Even the strongest person in the world would find it hard to deal with people continuously tearing them apart.

Someone slagging you off on Twitter is never okay. All you can do is try not to listen or take it to heart. You have to be mindful of the fact that they're just attacking an idea of you, and it often comes from jealousy and insecurity because you've got something they want. People who attack others on social media are bullies, pure and simple, so please ignore it as much as you can, and immediately block and report anyone who is bothering you. Sometimes someone will say something really horrible to me on Twitter and if I reply they'll say, 'Oh, thanks so much for replying!' The minute you stand up to bullies they back off. In a way you have to pity those people.

Don't think for one second that bullying just happens when you're a teenager or you work in an office. Bullying happens to me every day on social media and I completely understand how hard it can be to rise above it at times.

In the past when people called me bad things I'd believe what they said. I let them make me believe that I was 'famous for being vile on the telly' or I've 'got no friends'. I had to teach myself to be strong and block the negativity out. And I had to surround myself with good people whenever I could. I make sure I tell myself every day, over and over again, how much I believe in myself, and as a result most of those nasty remarks have become water off a duck's back. Please don't think I'm some kind of superhero who doesn't care about bad comments, because sometimes I really do. But I have got a hell of a lot better, and now blocking idiots on Instagram is one of my favourite hobbies!

In my opinion it's all about practice. You don't wake up one morning and suddenly feel strong. You have to work at it and convince yourself you're resilient until you're really there.

One thing I really want to say is this: don't believe everything you see. It's very easy for people to portray a certain image online, but please don't get hung up on social media. I know that's rich coming from me because I spend so many hours uploading pictures, replying to tweets and choosing the right filter, but essentially a lot of that is my job. And I try not to sit and stare at pictures of other people, wishing I had their life. Remember that very often social media isn't just about people editing pictures; they're editing their life. They're putting a Valencia filter on their *entire* life. And that's fine. Who cares? Why wouldn't you want to present the best image of yourself? Why wouldn't you want it to look like your life is incredible?

I would never knock someone for doing that, but at the same I would recommend that you try to keep some perspective. You've got the same filters that everyone else has got, and I bet they've got the same problems going on behind their filter as you have. Everything is not always all as it seems.

My Instagram may be full of pictures of me casually drinking smoothies, smashing it in the gym and having glamorous nights out with friends, but there are some mornings when I don't want to get out of bed. Or I'll have an argument with one of my friends and I'll feel so down and alone. And sometimes there are days when I even question if I'm doing the right thing with my life. Like everyone else, I have days where I sack the diet off entirely and eat a giant pizza. But those pictures never make the cut because I always try to put my game face on when it comes to presenting myself to the outside world.

Don't get hung up on the version of other people's lives they want you to see. Just because you don't see a photo of me in my holey pyjamas, scoffing a burger and crying because someone's written something horrible about me in a magazine, doesn't meant it doesn't happen sometimes. Look beyond the filter.

#nofilter

Going make-up free is a scary thing for lots of girls, and the ultimate confidence test. But I promise you it's really liberating!

I wanted to include this picture in *The Real Me* because this is the *real* me, stripped bare. I've never really minded people seeing me without a full face on, and now everyone's seen me all sweaty and make-up free in the jungle, I feel even more confident.

I quite often do it during the day because it's really good for your skin. If I don't have a photoshoot or I'm not on TV or having a big night out, I can guarantee you I won't be wearing make-up. As much as anything else, it's time consuming.

It's also nice to show another side of yourself to people, because then when you do make the effort and dress up people take a step back and they're like, *Whoa.* Rather than being glam and made-up all the time you can shock people. The juxtaposition of going bare faced and then full-on glamour is great. I don't mind being make-up free in front of a boyfriend either, and I happily do it when I go to the gym or go shopping.

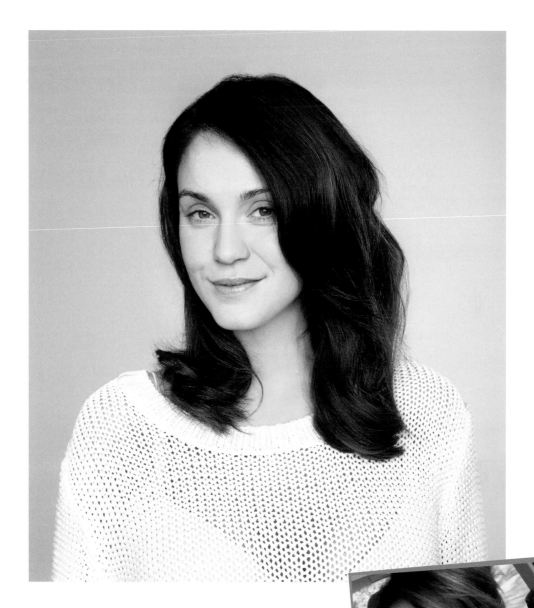

I suffer from spots sometimes but I don't think that's the end of the world. Everyone gets them now and again and I don't feel embarrassed about people seeing them if I'm not made up. Dare to bare! I think if you've got a decent set of HD eyebrows, a bit of a tan and some lip balm you look fine anyway. Embrace the natural you.

Some of my favourite memories from *I'm a Celebrity*. Did I mention I won?

This was the ultimate confidence test for me. Of course I was nervous about all the creepy crawlies and the trials, but there was also all the pressure I'd put on myself to do well.

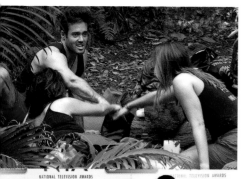

I'd wanted it for so long and I felt like this was my big chance to show the nation who I really was and what I could do, and I really didn't want to let myself down. Like most things though, the anticipation was the worst bit and once I actually got in there, I felt much more relaxed.

Walking into the jungle for the first time

What a moment! I'd watched the show for years and I was so excited about getting in there and getting cracking. I arrived by helicopter wearing a maxi dress and heels, but before you could say 'rice and beans' I was in my shorts, T-shirt and boots, raring to go. It was surreal actually arriving and meeting Spencer and Ferne, and then the rest of the camp, but it totally lived up to my expectations.

My fellow campmates

All the people I shared the jungle with were amazing. But as you'd expect, I got on with some people better than others. The only person I (briefly) fell out with was Yvette because one day she randomly accused me of pandering to Lady C and it annoyed me. She mistook my kindness for weakness but I soon put her right. She ended up apologising and it was all fine.

I learnt so much from my fellow campmates. Duncan has an amazing business brain and Chris taught me about sportsmanship, and Tony Hadley was a true gent. I was really lucky to have such a great group.

The trials

The trials were so much fun but Badvent Calendar and the Twister Tombola were my favourites. I felt like a warrior when I did them and I was determined to do well. I love a challenge and the trials taught me that I'm a real adrenaline junkie. Obviously I loved doing Cocktails and Screams and getting to drink camel peen too.

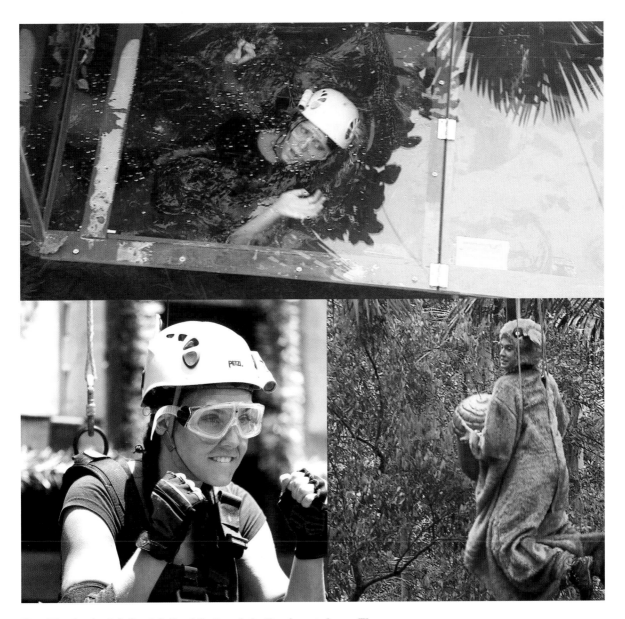

Top: *The final trial: Surf & Turf.* Bottom left: *Ready to take on The Badvent Calendar.* Bottom right: *Hanging around for The Nut Job.*

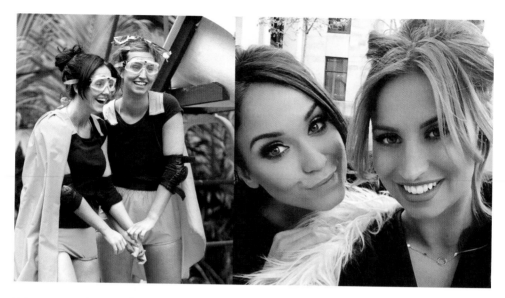

Becoming friends with Ferne

Everyone thought Ferne and I were going to be enemies because I'd once been on a date with her ex-boyfriend and she'd had some things to say about that in the press. To be fair, I kind of wondered whether we'd get on too. Whenever I saw her on *TOWIE* she was arguing with someone and I thought she was going to get on my nerves.

It was quite a weird dynamic because we had friends in common and we hung out at some of the same places, but we didn't actually know each other. But as everyone knows we hit it off straight away and she's became one of my best mates. The whole jungle experience was incredible, but she made it even better.

My bloody amazing three-course meal

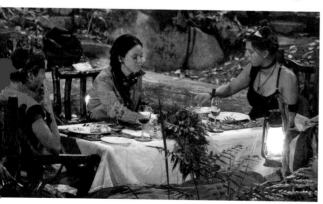

When George, Ferne and I won a three-course meal right near the end of the series it was like all my Christmases had come at once. We got to choose what we wanted and I went for a peperoni pizza followed by lasagne and chips and red velvet cake and vanilla ice-cream. I'm still furious I was too full to eat my dessert.

Winning!

I can't really explain how I felt when I found out I'd won. I honestly think that's the happiest I've ever been in my life. I was up against George Shelley and he said he didn't mind if he was didn't win because he was just happy to get to the final. I bloody wasn't – I wanted that crown!

The first thing what went through my head when my name was read out was, *Where's my mam?* It meant the world to me that I could finally make her proud after everything that had happened over the past few years. When I walked over the bridge and saw her it was almost too much and I burst into tears. I'll remember that moment as long as I live.

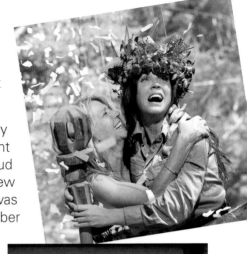

The after-party

I think the wrap party was when it really sank in that I'd won. The whole night was unbelievable. People were constantly coming up and congratulating me, and I had a real laugh with Ant and Dec. I even offered to get Kiosk Keith tequila – I think he thought I was trying to put a shift in. Come on Keith, man!

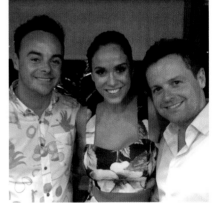

I celebrated like a true jungle queen and had to be carried out of the party afterwards. I felt that was my duty.

CELEBRATE GOOD TIMES!

How to throw the ultimate party.

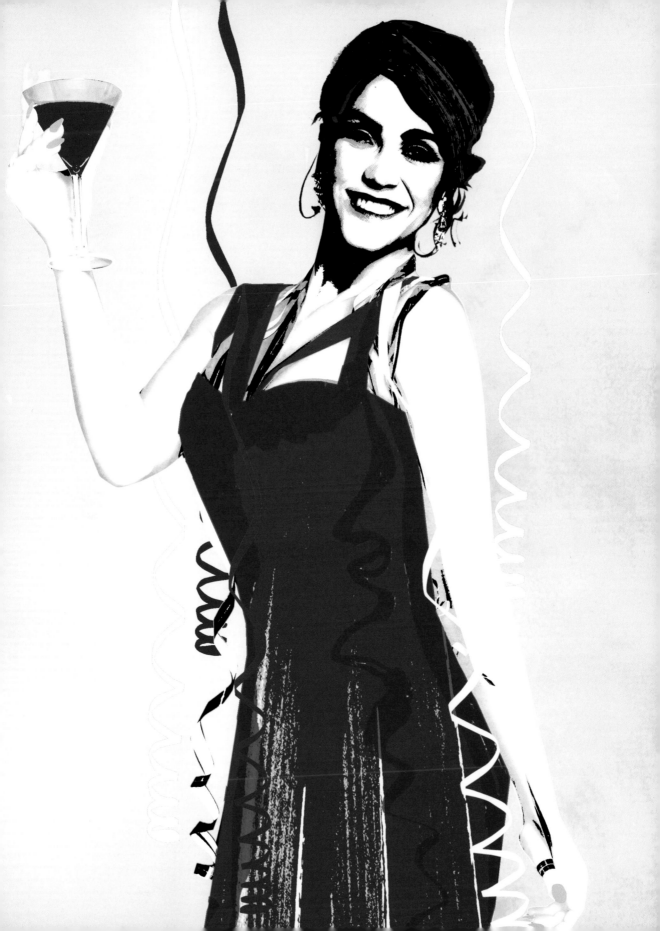

Who doesn't love a bloody good party?

I think it's pretty obvious that I'm the kind of girl who loves a party. I like throwing them, going to them, and recovering with a lot of beige food (sorry, I mean cleansing juices) *the following day. I've been to some amazing parties over the years, but I would say that my most memorable ones are . . .*

My 21st

I had a joint party with my friend Nicola and it was the girliest affair you've ever seen. It was a big hotel in Newcastle and the theme was cream, black and pink. I wore an Arrogant Cat dress and there was catering, themed cocktails, balloons, a three-tiered cake, speeches and a DJ. It was incredible and felt more like a royal wedding than a birthday to me.

All of my friends from school, uni and work came, and at the end of the night we rolled across the road to Liquid and Envy nightclub. It was all very swanks and I felt like a proper princess.

My friend Kailee's baby shower

Kailee was the first one of my friends to have a baby so it was a really big deal. I had everyone round to mine and because she was having a girl we had amazing pink and purple cocktails.

We had a gorgeous pink cake with an elephant on it, and this incredible Thai restaurant called Fat Buddha in Newcastle catered for it. We filled baby bottles with sweets so everyone had a party favour to take home. It was so lovely and perfect.

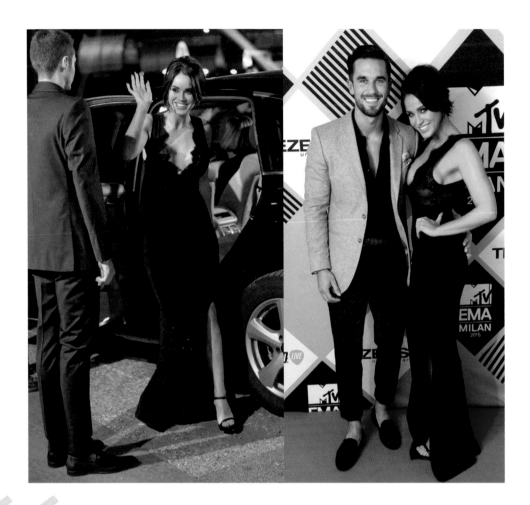

> **I'm not sure if anyone's ever danced around their handbag in Milan before so I think I lowered the tone.**

EMAs after-party in Milan

I went to the EMAs with Alex Cannon and we got *so* dressed up. People like Macklemore and Justin Bieber were flying about the party, and there was such a great atmosphere.

There was a free bar and live bands and Alex and I ended up dancing all night. I'm not sure if anyone's ever danced around their handbag in Milan before so I think I lowered the tone. We went home mortal drunk at 4 a.m. having had the best night ever.

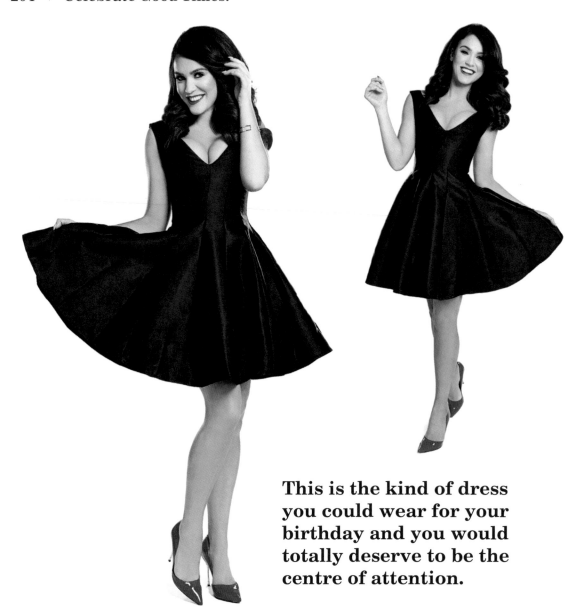

This is the kind of dress you could wear for your birthday and you would totally deserve to be the centre of attention.

Red-carpet glamour

Little black dresses are something every girl should have at least one of. This style is perfect for someone with my body shape. If you've got a big bum or thighs, skater skirts are gorgeous because they nip you in and then flare out. It skims over any lumps and bumps you might want to hide.

This dress has also got a great neckline so you can show a bit of cleavage. It's the perfect party dress and I feel like a dainty little doll and really sophisticated when I wear it, which is half the battle.

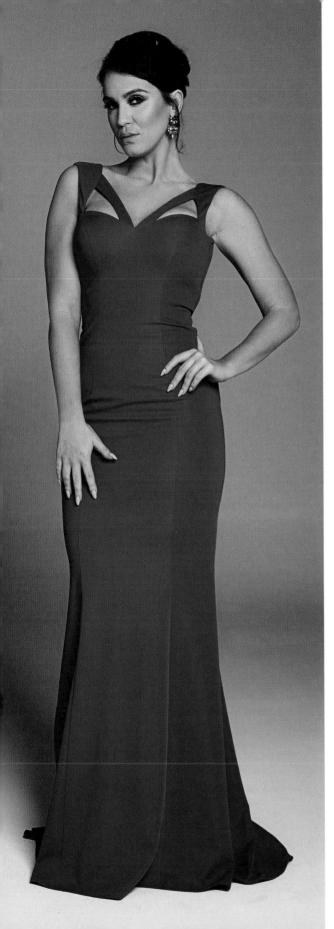

This dress would be amazing if you're going to a prom or a black-tie event. It's a perfect occasion dress.

Long dresses are always classy, and while they're not the most functional item of clothing in the world, they are worth the hassle because they look so good. The magenta colour is really different and it goes beautifully with gold.

There are two ways to go when it comes to what you wear under a dress this figure hugging. If you're feeling brave, you can wear nothing, and if you're not, go for shape underwear. I wore this dress in white for the NTAs earlier this year and I had nothing but a pair of nipple daisies underneath (I had no choice but to wear them. It was January and it was *very* cold). But there's so much amazing underwear available now, so that's always a great option. You can get corseted underwear, girdles, Spanx, slips, body stockings – you name it.

Please don't think tight dresses are only for the brave because there's something for everyone, and a dress this structured will help to hold you in anyway.

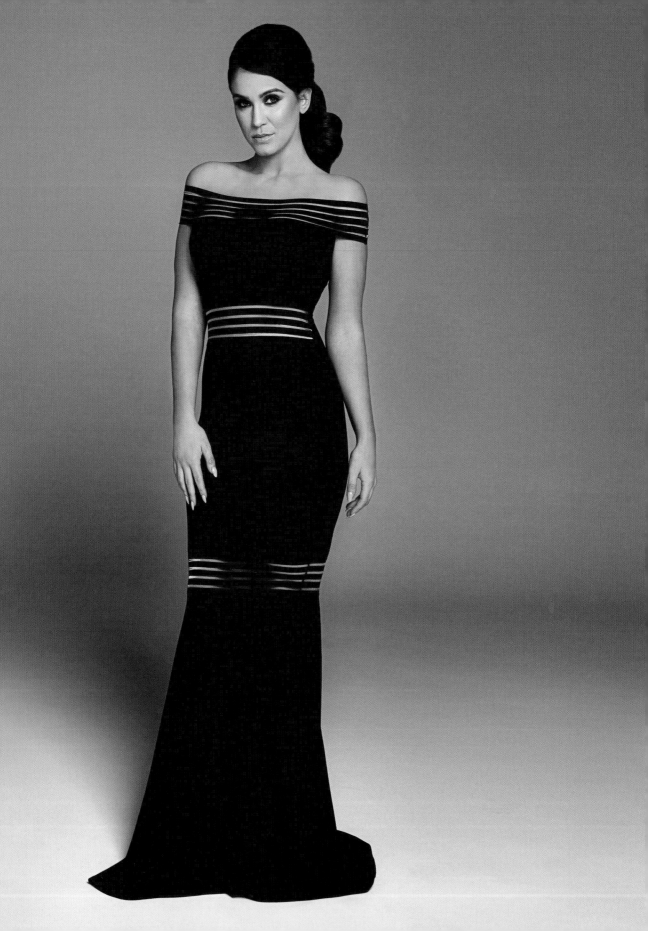

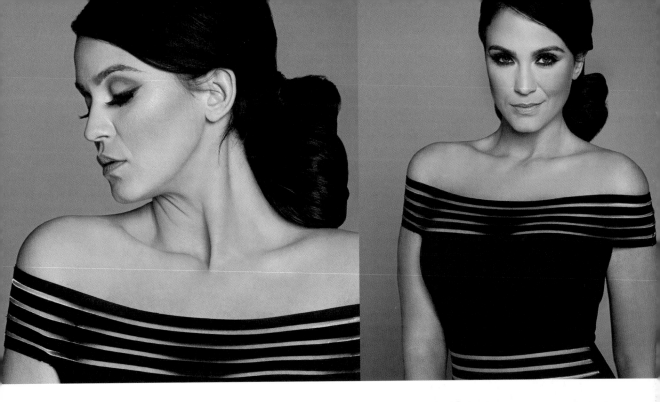

This dress is perfect for a spot of grocery shopping . . . or it may be more suited to a prom or a nice event! It's the type of thing you feel like a million dollars in. I think it's important for a girl to have at least one item like this in their wardrobe.

Black is slimming, sexy and classic. It's also one of the only colours that will go with any kind of accessory. This dress is also a prime example of quality not having to cost the earth. This little number is from Quiz but you could easily picture it on a Hollywood A-lister.

This totally suits my shape and the train is so decadent. I know a long train can be dangerous but just make sure it's not raining if you're going out in a full-length dress. I've fallen prey to that before and ruined a dress. I was going to a friend's birthday do and we weren't able to drive right up to the club. We had to walk a couple of hundred yards (my life can be so hard sometimes) and the pavement was soaking. By the time I got to the entrance the bottom of my beautiful green dress was wrecked. Because of that I made sure I got my NTAs dress altered to exactly the right length. If you're wearing something for a big occasion it's really worth spending the money on a good seamstress.

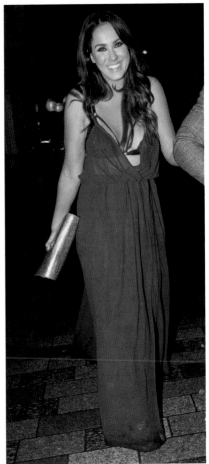

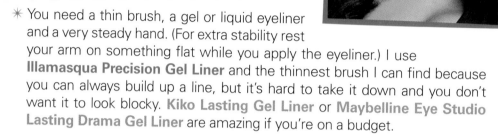

How to do flicked eyeliner like a pro

✳ Eyeliner is definitely easier to do on someone else, so you can always practise on friends before you do your own. This look is tricky to get right, and it really is a case of practice making perfect.

✳ You need a thin brush, a gel or liquid eyeliner and a very steady hand. (For extra stability rest your arm on something flat while you apply the eyeliner.) I use **Illamasqua Precision Gel Liner** and the thinnest brush I can find because you can always build up a line, but it's hard to take it down and you don't want it to look blocky. **Kiko Lasting Gel Liner** or **Maybelline Eye Studio Lasting Drama Gel Liner** are amazing if you're on a budget.

✳ It's better to keep eyes open when you're applying eyeliner because when they're closed your eyelids scrunch up, which isn't the best thing when you need a perfectly straight line!

✳ Start at the inner corner of your eye, and with the brush as close to the lash line as you can get, sweep along to the outer corner. It will take practice to be able to do it in one confident stroke, so you can start out doing it bit by bit and then going back to fill in any gaps you've missed. You'll find that the line naturally thickens as you get to the outer corner, which is ideal. Do this to both eyes.

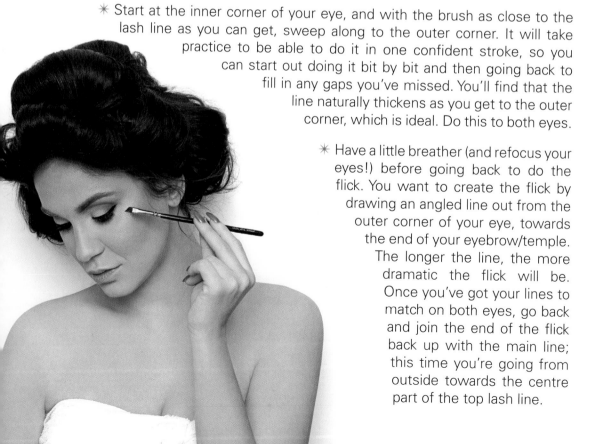

✳ Have a little breather (and refocus your eyes!) before going back to do the flick. You want to create the flick by drawing an angled line out from the outer corner of your eye, towards the end of your eyebrow/temple. The longer the line, the more dramatic the flick will be. Once you've got your lines to match on both eyes, go back and join the end of the flick back up with the main line; this time you're going from outside towards the centre part of the top lash line.

✳ Sometimes you'll find there isn't a tapered line or the line has a few bumps. This is easy to correct! Simply take a small eyeliner brush or cotton bud and dip in a non-oily eye make-up remover and apply. Repeat as many times as needed for a super clean liner.

✳ If you aren't confident about gel liner, you can always use a black or dark brown eyes shadow to create a smoky eyeliner rather than a defined flick. You can wet the brush when you want to move onto a more defined liner.

Quick up-do tips

Wearing your hair up for a special occasion always feels a bit more elegant, and if you've got a dress with an interesting neckline or you're wearing a statement necklace, it's a great way to make sure you show that off!

✳ I like to start by sectioning off my fringe. I don't like the look to be too polished – you don't want to look like a bridesmaid unless you actually are a bridesmaid! – so the idea is to have the fringe nice and sleek, but everything else a bit deliberately messy.

✳ I'll then backcomb my hair on top (as I do for the ponytail style on page 73) to give it height and get that sixties beehive vibe.

✳ Next I'll either pull the rest of my hair back into a ponytail then twist into a loose bun, securing with a few grips, or I'll just pin back random bits of hair and pin into place. You want it to be really textured, so don't pull anything back too tightly or worry about it all being really neat.

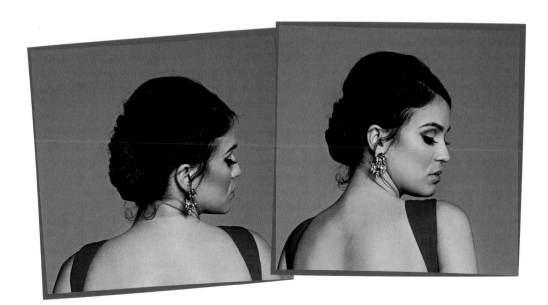

My Ultimate Party Playlist

Beautiful People by Chris Brown

Set You Free by N-Trance

Get Ugly by Jason Derulo

Freed from Desire by Gala

I Took a Pill in Ibiza by Mike Posner

Don't You Worry Child by Swedish House Mafia

In Da Club by 50 Cent

Sex on Fire by Kings of Leon

We Found Love by Rihanna featuring Calvin Harris

Sambuca (FooR remix) by Wideboys featuring Dennis G

Hey Mama by David Guetta and Nicki Minaj

Waiting for Love by Avicii

Rhythm is a Dancer by Snap

One Dance by Drake

This Is How We Do It by Montell Jordan

Light it Up by Major Lazer

I Predict a Riot by Kaiser Chiefs

Scandalous by Mystique

Where Are You Now by Justin Bieber

Let's Get it Started by Black Eyed Peas

Tips to help you throw the perfect party

* Commit. Throwing parties is sometimes stressful and difficult but you have to throw your whole self into it.

* Try not to get too stressed. Everyone will have an incredible time and it will be brilliant whether five or 105 people turn up, so just relax.

* Delegate. Don't put all the stress and pressure on yourself. Give people roles, like decorations or food, if they're happy to help out.

* Ask everyone to bring a bottle or some food, depending on the occasion. Make it a real group effort.

* Themed cocktails are always fun so embrace them. If it's someone's birthday you could do a cocktail with their favourite drinks in it and name it after them.

* Don't go overboard with the guest list because it can easily spiral out of control. More guests equals more money, so if in doubt just invite your nearest and dearest.

* Tell people they can have a plus one if they want one, especially if you know they won't know many other people. That way everyone will feel confident about mingling, which is what makes a party amazing.

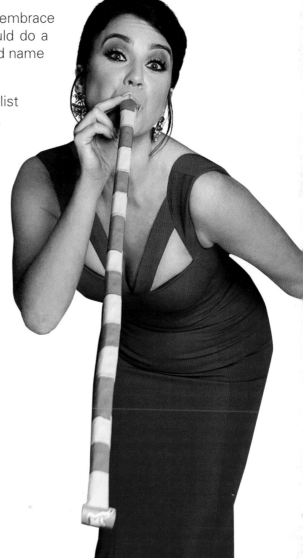

Commit. Throwing parties is sometimes stressful and difficult but you have to throw your whole self into it.

Peanut and coconut sauce with crudités

Impress your guests!

Ingredients

4 tablespoons peanut butter (use a good quality brand with no added sugar or salt)

1 handful of fresh coriander

1 fresh garlic clove

1 tablespoon soy sauce

Juice of 1 lime

4 tablespoons tinned coconut milk

1 tablespoon desiccated coconut (unsweetened)

½ teaspoon honey

Method

1. Simply place all the ingredients into a blender and process until smooth.

2. Store in a glass jar and keep refrigerated.

This works well as a dip for vegetables, or as a dipping sauce for mini chicken kebabs. Almond butter works well as a peanut butter substitute also.

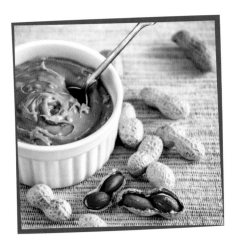

Benefits: *Peanut butter is a good source of vitamin E for healthy skin, and contains important vitamins and minerals for energy production, such as vitamin B3, B6, folate, magnesium and manganese.*

The fats in coconut milk are mainly medium-chain saturated fatty acids, which are easily converted to energy, and contain antiviral properties, to help boost your immune system.

'The Vicky' champagne cocktail

Ingredients

Peach purée
Juice of 1 lemon
1 bottle of rose water
Sugar syrup
1 bottle of pink
    Champagne

Method

1. Add 1 cup of peach purée to a mixing glass and add the lemon juice.

2. Add 4 tablespoons of rose water and 2 tablespoons of sugar syrup.

3. Muddle and mix together until the mixture is smooth and sieve through to another glass.

4. Pour chilled pink champagne into champagne flutes. Add the pre-made peach mixture to the flutes and garnish with rose petals!

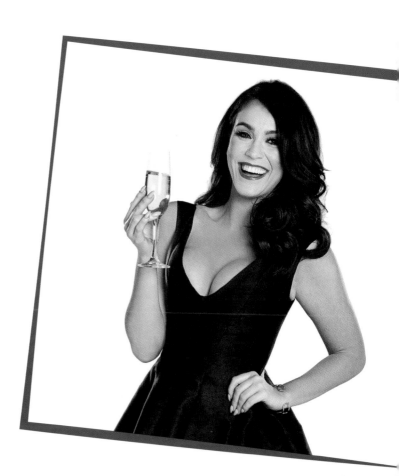

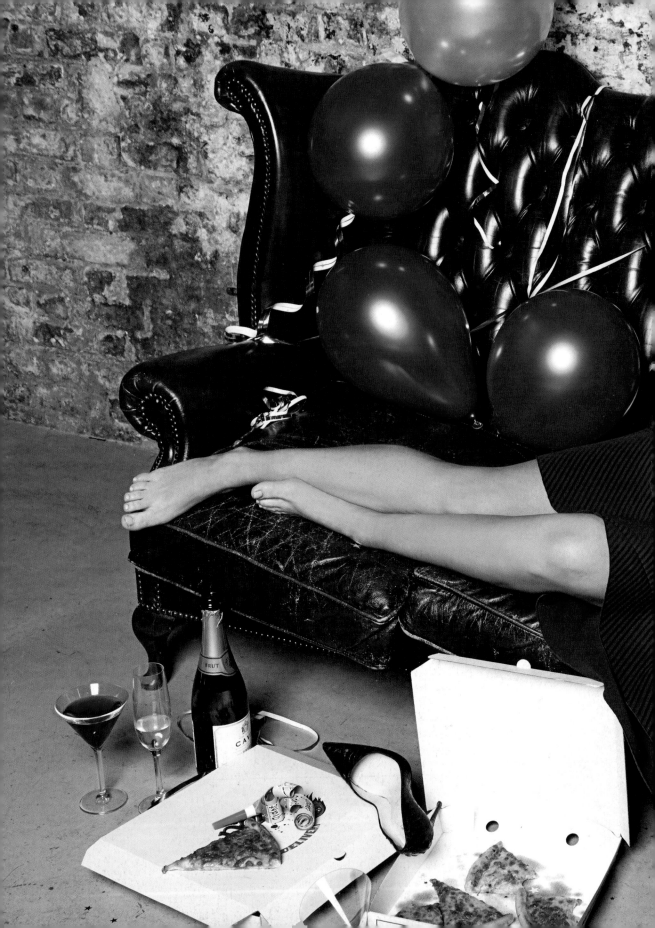

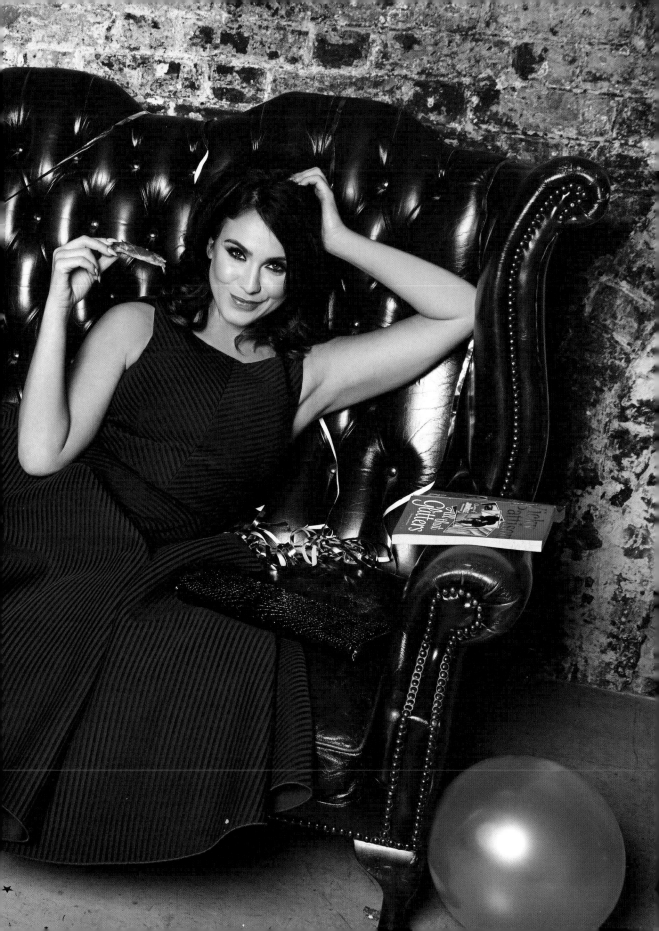

Bye for now . . .

Hi, and bye! I hope you've found this book useful and interesting. Maybe you've picked up some fashion tips or worked out a new hairstyle you like? Or maybe you've found exercising while you're working easier, or learnt a new way to deal with a break-up? Whatever it may be I hope you've taken something away from this book. It was a pleasure to work on and I'm really proud of it.

The last thing I want to say to everyone is that I truly believe if you have faith in yourself you can make anything happen. I'm a prime example of that.

When I first started on *Geordie Shore* I was £998 into my £1,000 overdraft limit, so I effectively had £2 to my name. I hardly earned any money, I didn't own a house and I had zero savings.

At that point I had no clue if the show would be a success, or what I'd do if it wasn't. I still didn't know what I wanted from my life. I just knew I wanted *something.*

I'd spent my last few quid on some clip-in hair extensions, and my mam took me shopping and bought me some clothes from Primark and TopShop so at least I had something new to wear in the house. Other than that, I was on my own embarking on an exciting but completely terrifying adventure.

When I look back at everything I've been through over the past seven years, it's been an interesting ride to say the least. There have been ups and downs, crap boyfriends and good ones, fat and slim days, a hideous court case, doubts, worries, triumphs . . . And when I look at where I am now, every single bit of it has been worth it.

The last thing I want to say to everyone is that I truly believe if you have faith in yourself you can make anything happen. I'm a prime example of that.

I'm a *Sunday Times* bestselling author, I've had a number one fitness DVD, I have a clothing company, a jewellery range and a fitness and nutrition brand. I write novels, I'm the Queen of the Jungle, I've got three hit MTV shows under my belt, I'm the youngest *Loose Women* panellist *ever*, I've got two houses, incredible friends and family, an amazing agent, and now I've written this book, which will go straight to the top of my achievement list. But most importantly, I have figured out how to do all of these by being *me*. The Real Me.

The future looks better than ever and I feel like the luckiest girl in the world. I believe in grafting hard, having a good time, training right, eating well and enjoying life. I believe in fate, destiny, luck and all of those things.

But more than anything, I believe in being grateful. So thank you to anyone who's read this book and supported me. It means the world to me and I hope it has helped you in some way.

All of my love,

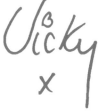

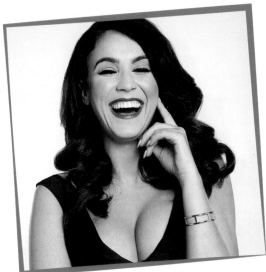

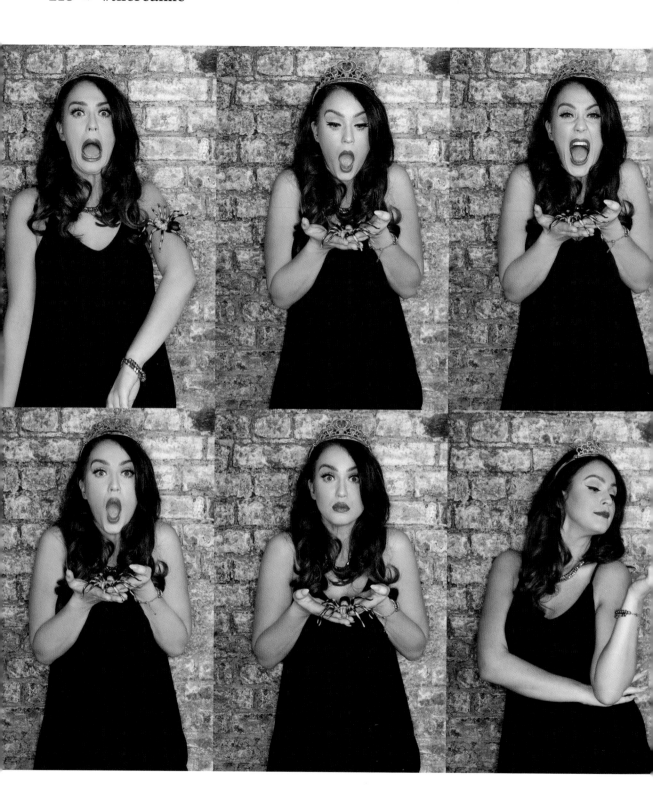

Acknowledgements

Firstly, thank you to my gorgeous Jordan Paramor. You know me better than I know myself these days, and I couldn't have done this without you.

THANK YOU to Sian and Emil from D.R. ink for all your hard work designing and laying out the whole book, but most importantly for those amazing hand-illustrated chapter-openers. Is it wrong that I want to wallpaper my new flat with them?

A massive shout-out to the whole creative crew who worked on the shoots: James and Georgia, Krystal, Chloe, Lo and Sarah. You're THE BEST. I love the shots so much, and I can't thank you enough. Extra love to Krystal and Chloe for all their help with the tutorials. And a special thank you to Linda Silverman from Little, Brown, who set up the shoots, kept the show on the road and tracked down pictures of me from all over the place!

Thanks to everyone at Motel Studios for looking after us so well on the shoots and letting me get pizza all over your nice sofa, and to my friends at my home-away-from-home, Park Plaza Hotels, for allowing us to shoot in one of your suites.

I also want to thank Brian Aris and Mikey Phillips for the additional photography in the book – especially the lovely central image on the cover.

So many people helped contribute to this book, and that includes Anthea, Nicky and the gang from Crush Cocktail Bars who all helped with recipes. Thank you so much!

Robbie Thompson, my patient and incredible personal trainer and friend – thank you for smashing it on the exercise programmes.

I'd love to thank everyone at Little, Brown for giving me the opportunity to continue working on brilliant books with them! But with special thanks to:

Hannah Boursnell for everything she's done to make this book possible and all her hard work and support on all my projects! Rachel Wilkie in marketing, Abby Marshall in production, Tracey Winwood for the gorgeous cover and all my friends in the sales team, who always support all my books so brilliantly – and always have biscuits when I stop by: Sara Talbot, Anna Curvis, Jen Wilson and Ben Goddard. Love to my amazing publicists Jo Wickham and Clara Diaz – and welcome to the squad, Ella Bowman. Can't wait to get The Real Me show on the road! Manpreet Grewal – my Mannaz! I'm buzzin' to start work on our next novel. And last but by no means least, thanks to the nicest big cheeses there are: David Shelley and Charlie King. You're the dream.

Thanks to my beautiful agents Gemma Wheatley and Nadia King, who saw something in me that no on else did and continue to work tirelessly to help me achieve my dreams.

My amazing sister and mother: you are everything to me and I couldn't live without you.

And finally, to everyone who has supported me and anyone who has ever bought one of my books . . . I love you all.

XXX

If you're making a recipe from *The Real Me* or trying one of the make-up tutorials – or you just want to shout about how amazing it is! – make sure you share your pictures and reviews with Vicky using **#therealme**. You can find her on Twitter **@vickygshore** and on Instagram **vicky_gshore**.

Contributors

Check out all the amazingly talented people who helped me with this book!

Design and illustration	**Emil Dacanay** and **Sian Rance** at D.R.ink | www.d-r-ink.com
Principal photography	**James Augustus** | www.jamesaugustusphotography.com
	🐦 @jamesaugustus74 | ⬜ jamesaugustus74
Photography assistant	**Georgia Shane** | ⬜ georgiashane
Stylist	**Sarah Cook** | www.sarahcookstylist.co.uk | ⬜ sarahcookstylist
Hair	**Chloe Oakes** | 🐦 @chloeoakes91
Make-up	**Krystal Dawn** | www.iammakeup.co.uk | ⬜ krystal_iammakeup
Additional hair and make-up	**Mikey Phillips** | www.makeupbymikey.com | ⬜ makeupbymikey
	Pages 42, 113, 122, 159, 162, 185, 187, 188
	Lo Dias | www.thebeautybom.com | ⬜ thebeautybom
	Pages 7, 27, 89, 91 (x2), 106 (x2), 108, 172, 182, 208
Additional photography	**Brian Aris** | www.brianaris.com
	Pages 42, 113, 122, 159, 162, 185, 187, 188
Recipes	**Anthea McCourtie** | www.younutritionaltherapy.co.uk
	🐦 @YouNutriTherapy | ⬜ YouNutritionalTherapy
	Pages 40, 75, 76, 77, 94, 100, 101, 102, 150 (nutritional advice), 173, 180, 181, 212
	Nicola Graimes | www.nicolagraimes.co.uk
	🐦 @NicolaGraimes
	Pages 61, 95, 108, 168
	Crush Cocktail Bars | www.crushcocktailbars.com
	🐦 @crushcocktail | ⬜ crushcocktailbars
	Pages 95, 109, 213
Exercise plans	**Robbie Thompson** | www.storm-fitness.com | 🐦 @robbiestormfit
	⬜ stormfitnesspt
Locations	**Motel Studios** | www.motelstudios.co.uk
	Park Plaza, County Hall | www.parkplaza.com/County-Hall

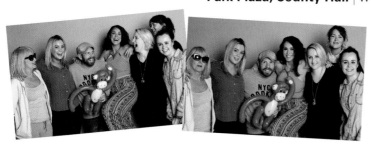

Linda, Chloe, James, Vicky, Jordan, Sarah and Hannah. Photos by Georgia Shane.

Picture credits

ANN SUMMERS
115; 132 (bottom)

BUMBLEBEE MEDIA
136 (bottom)

FAMEFLYNET.CO.UK
55; 207

GEMMA WHEATLEY
132 (top); 199 (bottom)

GETTY
30 (SamanthaJ/Getty Images); 51 (Karwai Tang/Getty Images); 65 (Neil Mockford/Getty Images); 82 (left; Barcroft Media/Getty Images); 86 (Mark Robert Milan/Stringer/Getty Images); 118 (Don Arnold/Getty Images) 203 (left; Gareth Cattermole/MTV 2015/Getty Images); 203 (right; Dave Hogan/MTV 2015/Getty Images)

iCELEB
24 (bottom); 57 (bottom)

INSTAGRAM/VICKY PATTISON
17; 21 (top); 21 (bottom); 24 (middle); 34; 82 (right); 101; 107; 123; 125; 174; 179; 195; 198 (right); 202 (bottom)

iSTOCK
76; 94; 100; 122; 150; 167; 168; 173; 180; 183; 191 (left); 191 (middle); 191 (right); 210; 212

JAMES RUDLAND/MOKKINGBIRD
78; 107; 137; 147; 169; 174; 190

KOBAL
103 (AMC/THE KOBAL COLLECTION)

PATTISON FAMILY/VICKY PATTISON
13 (top); 13 (middle); 13 (bottom); 14; 15 (top); 15 (bottom); 16; 44; 47; 49; 52; 164; 202 (top)

REX
53 (Palace Lee/REX/Shutterstock); 56 (Richard Young/REX/Shutterstock); 57 (top; Ken McKay/ITV/REX/Shutterstock); 73 (Ken McKay/ITV/REX/Shutterstock); 82 (middle; Palace Lee/REX/Shutterstock); 114 (Jonathan Hordle/REX/Shutterstock); 132 (middle; Graham Stone/REX/Shutterstock); 133 (Ken McKay/ITV/REX/Shutterstock); 136 (top; ITV/REX/Shutterstock); 153 (REX/Shutterstock); 154 (Nigel Wright/REX/Shutterstock); 178 (REX/Shutterstock); 196 (top; ITV/REX/Shutterstock); 196 (bottom; David Fisher/REX/Shutterstock); 197 (top; ITV/REX/Shutterstock); 197 (bottom left; ITV/REX/Shutterstock); 197 (bottom right; ITV/REX/Shutterstock) 198 (top left; ITV/REX/Shutterstock); 198 (bottom; ITV/REX/Shutterstock) ; 199 (top; ITV/REX/Shutterstock); 203 (Richard Isaac/REX/Shutterstock)

SHUTTERSTOCK
41; 75 (top); 75 (bottom)

WENN.COM
26

XPOSURE.COM
24 (Timms/Xposurephotos.com)

Fashion credits

Thank you so much to everyone who kindly provided clothes for the book!

Page 9
Blue asymmetric dress by Quiz

Pages 29–31
✳ Black and red 'VIP Privileged' dress and red clutch by VIP Collection by Vicky Pattison for Honeyz; shoes Vicky's own
✳ Shirt-dress 'VIP Bow Shirt' by VIP Collection for Honeyz; faux suede boots by Quiz; Prada handbag, Vicky's own
✳ Denim dress by H&M; faux suede jacket by Zara; boots by Mango; handbag, Vicky's own
✳ Pink and white 'VIP Elle'Lee Skirt', white 'VIP Paparazzi Top' and white 'VIP Heels' by VIP Collection for Honeyz

Page 69
✳ Coat-dress 'VIP Belted Gridlock Dress' by VIP Collection for Honeyz; red shoes and Prada handbag, Vicky's own

Page 72
✳ White shirt and 'VIP 3 Way MAC Jacket' by VIP Collection for Honeyz; navy culotte jumpsuit by Limited Collection at Marks & Spencer; shoes, Vicky's own

Pages 86–7
✳ Orange and pink 'VIP Colour Crush' dress by VIP Collection for Honeyz; purple shoes, Vicky's own
✳ Red skirt and stripy top 'VIP Famous Co/Ord' by VIP Collection for Honeyz
✳ White dress by River Island; gold bangles by Chained & Able; gold shoes and YSL clutch, Vicky's own

Page 88
✳ Yellow jumpsuit by River Island; earrings, stylist's own; blue shoes, Primark. (Ring courtesy of Manpreet Grewal – thanks, Mannaz!)

Page 98
✳ Lounge wear by TopShop

Page 151
✳ Grecian dress by House of CB; necklace by Chained & Able

Page 152–3
✳ 'VIP Yellow Obsession' dress by VIP Collection for Honeyz; gold shoes, Vicky's own
✳ Black maxi 'VIP Luxe Lounge' dress by VIP Collection for Honeyz; gold necklace and earrings by Souksy; gold bangles by Chained & Able; sandals by New Look
✳ Orange top and Palazzo pants 'VIP Bold and Beautiful Co/Ord' by VIP Collection for Honeyz; necklace by Souksy; wedges by New Look; sunglasses, stylist's own

Page 155
✳ Tanning onesie by Bronzie

Page 204–5
✳ Black dress by Girl In Mind; red shoes, Vicky's own
✳ Purple floor-length dress by Pia Michi, earrings by Souksy

Page 206
✳ Black floor-length dress by Quiz

Stockists
www.honeyz.com
www.newlook.com
www.hm.com
www.riverisland.com
www.girlinmind.com
www.zara.com
www.mango.com
www.quizclothing.co.uk
www.chainedandable.com
www.souksy.com
www.piamichi.com
www.topshop.com
www.bronzieuk.com
www.marksandspencer.com
www.houseofcb.com

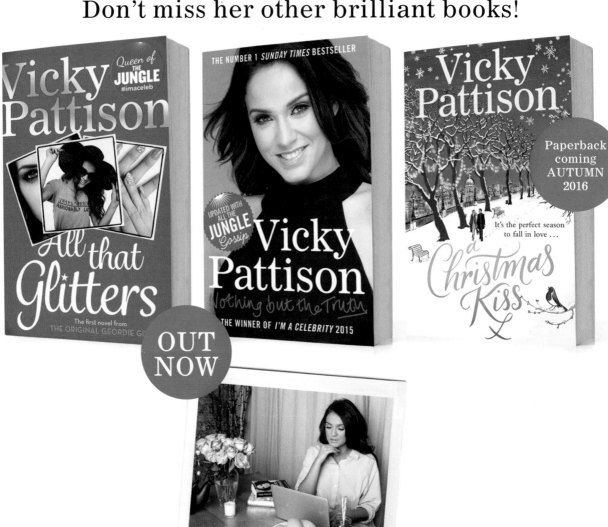